MAN FOR MAN

**A Multidisciplinary Workshop on Affecting
Man's Social and Psychological Nature
Through Community Action**

MAN FOR MAN

**A MULTIDISCIPLINARY WORKSHOP ON AFFECTING
MAN'S SOCIAL AND PSYCHOLOGICAL NATURE
THROUGH COMMUNITY ACTION**

Edited by

JOHN L. CARLETON, M.D.

Founder, Santa Barbara Psychiatric Medical Group

and

URSULA MAHLENDORF, Ph.D.

Associate Professor
Department of Germanic and Slavic Languages and Literature
University of California, Santa Barbara

CHARLES C THOMAS · PUBLISHER
Springfield · Illinois · U.S.A.

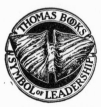

Published and Distributed Throughout the World by

CHARLES C THOMAS • PUBLISHER

Bannerstone House

301-327 East Lawrence Avenue, Springfield, Illinois, U.S.A.

© *1973, by* CHARLES C THOMAS • PUBLISHER

ISBN 0-398-02754-4

Library of Congress Catalog Card Number: 72-93203

With THOMAS BOOKS careful attention is given to all details of
manufacturing and design. It is the Publisher's desire to present books that are
satisfactory as to their physical qualities and artistic possibilities and
appropriate for their particular use. THOMAS BOOKS will be true to those
laws of quality that assure a good name and good will.

Printed in the United States of America

H-2

DEDICATION

THIS BOOK is dedicated to those who support and devote their lives to our endeavor—may the light from this candle combine with that from a billion more to make this earth a better place to live.

CONTRIBUTING AUTHORS

Steve Allen. Television Commentator; Motion Picture Actor; Musician; Author; Producer; Poet and Documentarian.

Alfred Auerback, M.D. Clinical Professor of Psychiatry at University of California Medical Center, San Francisco; Chairman of the San Francisco Mental Health Advisory Board; Past President Northern California Psychiatric Society; Past Vice-President American Psychiatric Association.

Joshua Bierer, M.D., D. Econ. and Soc. Sc. Medical Director of the Institute for Social Psychiatry; Editor of *International and British Journals of Social Psychiatry;* Founder of Marlborough Hospital; Chairman, International Association of Social Psychiatry; (London, England).

Daniel Blain, M.D. Director, Philadelphia State Hospital. Past President American Psychiatric Association; Past Medical Director American Psychiatric Association; Past Director Department of Mental Hygiene, State of California (1959-1963).

C. H. Hardin Branch, M.D. Assistant Director, Santa Barbara County Mental Health Services. Past Professor and Head of Department of Psychiatry, University of Utah; Past President American Psychiatric Association; President American Board of Psychiatry and Neurology.

Norman Q. Brill, M.D. Professor and Past Chairman, Department of Psychiatry, Neuropsychiatric Institute, UCLA; Consultant, Office Surgeon General, Department Army, Navy, Air Force; Chairman American Psychiatric Association Council on Professions.

John L. Carleton, M.D. Founder, Santa Barbara Psychiatric Medical Group; Psychiatrist in Private Practice; Secretary, American Association for Social Psychiatry.

Luba F. Carleton, B.A. Educational Therapist, Santa Barbara

Psychiatric Medical Group; Special Education Teacher, Santa Barbara City School District; Member, Board of Directors, Santa Barbara Psychiatric Foundation.

Price M. Cobbs, M.D. Assistant Clinical Professor of Psychiatry, University of California Medical Center, San Francisco; Director, Racial Confrontation Group Project, San Francisco Medical Center, University of California; Consultant to Executive Development Program National Urban League; Private Practice; Co-Author of *Black Rage;* Author *The Jesus Bag*, March, 1971.

Erika Freeman, Ed.D. Professor of Social Psychiatry, Sarah Lawrence; Vice-president and Co-founder of International Association of Study of Group Tension; Personal Advisor to United Nations Interregional Director for Youth Programs of Developing Nations; Political Psychoanalyst.

Harry Girvetz, Ph.D. Professor of Philosophy, University of California, Santa Barbara; Editor, *Science, Folklore, and Philosophy;* Author, *Democracy and Elitism;* "Liberalism," Encyclopedia Britannica; Research Secretary to Governor Pat Brown.

Frank K. Kelly. Vice-president Center for the Study of Democratic Institutions; Speechwriter for President Truman; Author, *The Fight for the White House; Men Who Make Your World; Your Laws;* Proposer of Annual Report on the State of Mankind; National Board of Director of the National Book Committee.

Dan R. Kennedy, M.A. Minister at University Methodist Church of Goleta and Campus Pastor at UCSB; Co-founder and Director of *The Openings*, a retreat and human resources center; Elected Member Isla Vista Community Council.

Burton Kerish, M.A. Clinical Psychologist, U.S.P.H.S. Federal Bureau of Prisons; Psychologist in Private Practice.

Frank Lanterman. California Legislator; Co-author Lanterman-Petris-Short Act; Assemblyman Fourth District; Author California Mental Retardation Act; Past Chairman and Current Vice-Chairman of Ways and Means Committee.

Ursula R. Mahlendorf, Ph.D. Associate Professor, Department of Germanic and Slavic Languages and Literatures, University of California, Santa Barbara. President, Psychiatric Foundation of Santa Barbara.

Norbert J. McNamara, M.D. Director, Santa Barbara County Mental Health Services; Consultant to NASA; Consultant to Department of Labor Manpower Administration.

Louis Miller, M.D. Chief National Psychiatrist and Director of Mental Health Services, the State of Israel; Vice Chairman International Association for Social Psychiatry; Editor of *Mental Health in Rapid Social Change;* Member, Executive Committee, World Federation for Mental Health.

Louis J. Rozenfeld. Architect; Chief Planner and Manager of Community Planning and Regional Development for the Bechtel Corporation; responsibility for planning and environment projects throughout the world.

J. B. Tietz, LL.B. Draft and Military Law since 1944; has argued over one hundred federal appellate draft cases, including Welsh vs United States 90 S.Ct. 1792 (1970) regarding conscientious objectors to war.

PREFACE

D URING MOST of 1969 and 1970, the Executive Committee of the newly reorganized International Association of Social Psychiatry formulated plans for a number of international meetings and professional activities. The Santa Barbara Social Psychiatry Workshop, which was held in March of 1971, is an outgrowth of this planning. Preceding our workshop, there occurred under the leadership of Jules H. Masserman, M.D., the First International Soviet-American Symposium on Social Psychiatry which was held in Moscow and Leningrad, Russia; Budapest, Hungary; and Dubrovnik and Zagreb, Yugoslavia, in September of 1970. Immediately following that meeting, the Third International Congress of Social Psychiatry, organized primarily by Doctor Vladimir Hudolin, M.D., of Zagreb, was held in Zagreb, Yugoslavia, September 21 to 26, 1970. The Santa Barbara Workshop was planned by Joshua Bierer, M.D. and John L. Carleton, M.D. during the week following the International Congress.

The primary purpose of the International Association of Social Psychiatry and its component divisional groups, including the American Association for Social Psychiatry, is humanitarian. Social psychiatric principles have now reached that state of development and validation at which they can realistically be incorporated into all aspects and facets of human existence. On a philosophical level, these principles facilitate the understanding of intrapsychic functioning and they also offer new insights into all interpersonal relationships.

Those who are familiar with these principles and who have been involved in their development and evolution are not only committed to the further development and evolution of the principles but are convinced that they offer a very important and necessary contribution to the cause of peace for all mankind.

Dr. Thomas Rennie, M.D., in an article of the first issue of *The International Journal of Social Psychiatry* in 1955, stated that

"Social psychiatry is etiological in its aim, but its point of attack is the whole social framework of contemporary living."[1] In his presidential address to the American Psychiatric Association in May of 1957, Dr. Francis J. Braceland stated,

> The psychiatrist in research and in practice is not justified in restricting his endeavors to one aspect of the human being. He has to take account of man as a whole, and in the totality of his vital, social, cultural situation. Paradoxical though it may sound, the statement is nonetheless cogent, that to be truly a psychiatrist, one has to be more than a psychiatrist, more than a specialist. . . . While scientific enquiry and methodology must always form the solid foundation of our discipline, upon this foundation may be erected the edifice of a psychiatry which will be the "applied science of man."[2]

Dr. Joshua Bierer has many times called for the development of a *multidisciplinary science* for the study of man. Thus, it is entirely appropriate that a multi-disciplinary orientation was adopted for the March 1971 Santa Barbara Workshop, and that this orientation applied to all participants, whether they were at the podium or in the audience. This proved to be a very successful and rewarding orientation. A very warm and cohesive spirit developed between all who attended the relatively short meeting. Although many participants at the outset of the workshop were not aware that psychiatric patients manned the registration desk, helped to set up the meetings, taped the sessions, and served as hosts and hostesses at the luncheon interaction groups, it was these patients' involvement which contributed directly to the openness and comfort of the conference milieu.

In addition to the presentations at the workshop, several other papers have been added to this volume. The first paper by Dr. Daniel Blain concerns the last twenty-five years of American Psychiatry and provides an excellent historical and informative background in which American Social Psychiatry has many of its roots. The paper by Dr. Louis Miller concerning violence and group identity is an important addition to the international concerns of the workshop and strengthens considerably that dimension of this volume. Dr. Miller's paper is the result of a vast and personal experience in Israel whose recent growth is in itself an amazing example of social development.

That this development should take place in an area which is, for Western Civilization, *the origin,* is even more significant. At an opposite extreme, though certainly no less significant and valuable, is the paper by Dr. Ursula Mahlendorf, vice-president and currently president, of the Psychiatric Foundation of Santa Barbara. She has written about her own therapy and more specifically about her involvement with clay modelling and wood sculpturing as a part of her total experiential therapy. Luba Carleton's paper reports on the social and human interaction during the workshop and describes many of the behind-the-scenes activities without which the workshop would not have been. Her paper involves the soul of the workshop and concerns many aspects, including the participation of the patients and the personal and social activities without which collaboration is impossible anywhere. For these activities are as important, if not more so, than the more masculine and intellectual utterances of the panelists and speakers. Both masculine and feminine components are equally necessary to the achievement of the stated goals of this workshop.

It is the hope of all of us who participated that those of you who read these pages will catch some of the spirit of which we speak as well as find new insights and new directions for the future.

We extend great appreciation to the participant audience and to the speakers for their extremely valuable contributions. We sincerely thank the University of California Extension at Santa Barbara, and George H. Daigneault, Ph.D., Dean of the Extension and Mrs. Betty L. Harris, Program Representative, University Extension, for organizing and arranging the academic aspects of the workshop.

Generous financial support was provided by Geigy Pharmaceuticals, Merck, Sharp and Dohme, Roche Laboratories and Mr. and Mrs. John Mealy. Because of this support, many students were able to receive scholarships to attend the workshop. Mr.

Robert Brown, President of the Psychiatric Foundation of Santa Barbara and John Mealy, technical advisor for the workshop deserve special mention for their contribution and effort. Members of the Santa Barbara Psychiatric Medical Group, especially Joan Smallwood, dance therapist and Elaine Pedigo, social worker are to be remembered for their devotion before, during and after the workshop and for their contribution to its content and organization; Judith Krayk, our secretary for providing the support and services which only a secretary can do.

The preparation of the manuscript would have been impossible without the diligent assistance of Kathlyn Stentz, who proofread and typed the final draft. Additional back-up support was provided by Robin Hamlin, Jennie Brown and my daughter Bari. Ursula Mahlendorf, the co-editor, has given endless hours to her task. We extend gratitude and appreciation for her fine job and for her continuing moral support in the endeavor.

We gratefully acknowledge the permission to reprint the following two contributions: To the *Israel Annals of Psychiatry and Related Disciplines* for Louis Miller's essay *Identity and Violence*. To Littlefield, Adams and Company for permission to reprint *An Anatomy of Violence*, as it is to appear in their forthcoming volume *Reason and Violence*, edited by Sherman Stanage, Ph.D., Littlefield, Adams and Company, Totowa, New Jersey, 1972. We also wish to express appreciation to B. E. McLaughlin, M.D., Medical Director of Calabasas Hospital for permission to print Daniel Blain's contribution.

Finally, to my wife Luba a special kind of appreciation is due because it was she who was the catalyst and crystallized the effort and the spirit which gave the workshop life.

JOHN L. CARLETON, M.D.

BIBLIOGRAPHY

1. Rennie, Thomas A. C.: Social Psychiatry—A Definition. *The International Journal of Social Psychiatry*, 1(1):12, 1955.
2. Psychiatry and the Science of Man: In *New Directions in American Psychiatry 1944-1968*. American Psychiatric Association, Washington, D.C., 1969, p. 173.

WELCOMING

G OOD MORNING, ladies and gentlemen. My name is Bob Brown.
As president of the Psychiatric Foundation of Santa Barbara,
I would like to welcome you this morning to our workshop. We
have some very distinguished guests and speakers and a most interesting program; I am sure you will enjoy participating in it. I
would like to take a few minutes at this time to tell you something about our foundation.

It was about in June of last year when a group of us got together to discuss some of the problems of mental health here in Santa
Barbara. Because of our own experiences, we felt we knew what
many of the problems confronting the psychiatric patients were.
Our group consisted of patients, relatives of patients, therapists
and other professional people. In the group we had one very
strong common belief; that belief was that an individual should
have the right and the opportunity to experience his feelings and
to be able to express these feelings openly and honestly without
fear of rejection or retribution by others. This is pretty easy to
say, but very difficult to do.

The initial task we wanted to undertake as a group was that of
providing assistance to people who were about to leave the psychiatric ward of the hospital and return to their homes, their
responsibilities in the home and their responsibilities in the outside world of society. We felt that if we could provide an emotionally supportive community in which the patient could live
for an interim period, we could help him to handle his problems
better when he did return home. The more we thought about
this problem the more realistic it became that we could and
should try to do something. We decided to go ahead with the
plan; the plan was that we would locate a house suitable for
this purpose. We would also establish a nonprofit foundation to
handle the business affairs of running a half-way house.

Working together, we all put ourselves into the project and

we soon found the house we were looking for. Work parties developed spontaneously, and we prepared, cleaned, and painted the house. Other people located and got furniture and furnishings for the house. All of this happened and got completed so fast that it was really hard to believe. After we got through with this phase of the work, we had a party, inviting all the people involved in the project. The warmth that came from that group of people I personally had never experienced before, and I was really glad to be a part of it. There were a lot of people investing their time, their effort, and their money, but I think most important of all, they invested themselves. They were involved. The interaction that went on among the people was hard to believe.

The basic concept that we wanted the community to establish and to maintain was to base the community on honesty and openness with one another and above all, on love for one another. As individuals and as a group we achieved that. It wasn't long before the house was occupied. The community was self-governing and all the decision-making processes were made by the residents of the community. The people living at the house supported one another in meeting new challenges and new responsibilities in the outside world and in their community itself. They learned to relate to each other and to other people. The more supportive they were of each other, the more comfortable they became with expressing their feelings and with overcoming the fear of rejection in doing so. Some of the problems they faced they handled with relative ease, but others were very difficult for them. They had to handle the problems of working out feelings about each other and about themselves; they did this with each other, which is difficult to do. The feelings of anger and hostility are always hard to deal with. But there were good feelings that were difficult for them to deal with also. The fear of being close to one another, to be exposed, to expose yourself to other people—these things they had to handle, and they did handle them. The important thing was that they faced the problems and got through them to a conclusion.

They were establishing and controlling their environment. The more comfortable the people became with themselves and with

each other, the more they were able to accept additional responsibilities and to become involved in newer things, bigger
things. They began to bring the outside world into their community, thereby expanding their world and realizing more fully
their individual potentials. They were growing and their world
was growing with them. They began to schedule regular evenings
for open house, and members of the foundation, friends, and
relatives would drop by. Sometimes they would just sit around
and talk, express their ideas and their views and opinions, express and share their feelings about themselves and about one
another. Sometimes a group would sit on the floor and carve
wood or work in pottery. But all of these things were an expression of the people involved. The closeness among the people involved continued to grow. They became closer and closer. It got
to the point—this is my feeling, and I am sure a feeling most of
the other people involved share—it got to the point where everyone became a member of one large family. That family, because
of the love within it, supplied many of the needs for emotional
support, that is, honest criticism and assistance. It supplied
structure where it was needed and the lack of structure where
that was needed. It gave encouragement that each member could
accomplish what he wanted to accomplish as an individual.
They could overcome the problems they were facing every day.
Once again, they did this and they are still doing it.

It has been a very rewarding experience for me personally to
be involved and to see the growth in other people as well as the
growth within myself. I think that this stems primarily from being
a part of this family. It has been good to be a part of it, and I
certainly intend to remain a part of it. You see, our family believes, as you people believe, in what we are doing. We believe
that the only thing that makes anything else worth while is the
people. That's where it is and that is where it has got to stay.
Our involvement in sponsoring this workshop today is an illustration of our beliefs and of our continuing growth as people.
Ladies and gentlemen, your interest and your participation by
being here today is indicative of where we are going in the future.
For those of you who might be interested and would like to drop

by, we are having open house at our half-way house this evening
between the hours of 7:30 and 9:30. If you would like to drop
by, you can get additional information at the registration desk
anytime today. I'll be looking forward to seeing some of you
there.

ROBERT G. BROWN

OPENING REMARKS

I AM MOST IMPRESSED with Bob Brown's remarks this morning and really so thrilled with them that I think if we hear no more, we've already heard the best of the program. Thank you very much, Bob.

Among some people there is an ever-increasing awareness of the necessity for a coordinated, multidisciplinary approach to the problems which beset mankind. Joshua Bierer, our principal speaker, has called for the formation of a multidisciplinary science to facilitate that approach. Vital and integral to this idea is the capacity to maintain a global perspective when analyzing any human problem. Social psychiatry is the natural, evolutionary evolvement of psychiatry because it directs itself to the whole person and utilizes information from every possible source when attempting to solve a person's behavioral problems.

Social psychiatry, the designation which I believe best covers this global approach, is a multidisciplinary science. Traditionally, the psychiatrist, a medical doctor, has concerned himself with the manifestations of *mental illness*. We shall learn from Doctor Bierer that there is grave question about the validity of our current diagnostic practices and nomenclature for mental illness.[1] Others have also strongly criticized these practices.[2] Certainly ever-increasing awareness that family, parents, siblings, groups, national identities, international realities, war, poverty, energy needs, pollution and racism have a direct influence upon the etiology and manifestations of emotional illness and social conduct compels the modern psychiatrist to expand his horizons sufficiently to encompass these facts before he labels his patient with a diagnostic tag. A boil, is not, although it relates to, the entire person. Social behavior, emotional reactions and psychic phenomena, are however, manifestations of the global experiences of the human being.

A traditional medical model cannot meet the needs of our developing science of social psychiatry. Attitudes, prejudices, expectations, cultural influences, relative degrees of predictability of the milieu and a multitude of additional factors must be considered during the diagnostic process. It is not correct to label a person as a *manic depressive* for example. It is only possible to describe or predict the probable behavioral or psychic manifestations of an individual given a certain set of experiences and circumstances. Each person must be considered individually in the light of his own biological realities and social experiences and we must avoid the diagnostic nihilism of believing that a statistical diagnostic tag is anything more than an attempt to describe a part of a reaction pattern.

Those life experiences which compel individuals to become alcoholic, drug abusers, fanatical dictators, unscrupulous businessmen, self-seeking politicians, criminals, or mentally ill are social in nature. Venereal disease may be a medical illness in the vagina, but its prevention is a social problem. War is a social psychiatric problem and so are the personal motivations which lead to corruption in government.

Objective, effective utilization of the factual insights gained from millions of hours of psychotherapeutic research is an essential necessity if governments, corporations, people are to solve their most difficult problems, those of living and surviving together. Social psychiatrists must prepare themselves to function as advisors to political leaders, corporate board chairmen, judges, attorneys, presidents, governors, mayors and supervisors. The latter must prepare themselves to be receptive of such counsel. Humanitarianism must become the by-word for all social interaction. To prepare himself for such advisory capacities, the social psychiatrist must understand more and more about the other disciplines, sciences, professional activities, philosophies and groups which contribute to and have such a profound impact upon the human being. It is with these ideas in mind that the discussions in which you will participate during the next three days were organized.

I believe they will make a significant step and contribution to the science of social psychiatry.

JOHN L. CARLETON

BIBLIOGRAPHY

1. Bierer, Joshua: The Validity of Psychiatric Diagnosis. *The International Journal of Social Psychiatry,* 1(1):22-30, 1955.
2. Cf. Menninger, Karl: Syndrome, Yes; Disease Entity, No. In Cancro, Robert (Ed.): *The Schizophrenic Reactions: A Critique of the Concept, Hospital Treatment, and Current Research.* New York, Brunner-Mazel, 1970, pp. 71-78.

CONTENTS

Part I

U.S. PSYCHIATRY

Part II

SOCIAL PSYCHIATRY

Part III

PLANNING FOR THE MENTAL HEALTH OF THE COMMUNITY

Part IV

CONTEMPORARY SOCIAL PROBLEMS

Part V

NATIONS AND COMMUNITIES: TOWARD
A HEALTHY WORLD

Part VI

EXPERIENTIAL THERAPY

MAN FOR MAN

**A Multidisciplinary Workshop on Affecting
Man's Social and Psychological Nature
Through Community Action**

PART I
U.S. PSYCHIATRY

Chapter 1

U.S. PSYCHIATRY, 1972: WHERE ARE WE NOW, WHERE ARE WE GOING?*

DANIEL BLAIN, M.D.

INTRODUCTION
John L. Carleton, M.D.

Dr. Blain is uniquely qualified as a discussant of the past twenty-five years in American psychiatry. His personal participation and continuous involvement have given him a perspective which most of us could not have, yet such a perspective is vitally important to the understanding of the present and future of our field of endeavor. Dr. Blain has, if you will, "grown up in American psychiatry." With Freud, Bleuler and Meyer as his "fathers," he has had a unique experience. He has seen the developments in psychiatry grow and evolve from the confined and limited sphere of "intrapsychic or intrapersonal" to the current rapidly growing concern for the "world around the patient." In other words he has seen psychiatry's growth from an almost total commitment to the individual to community psychiatry as we know it today. His training included psychoanalysis and his perspective is truly that of a social psychiatrist.

Dr. Daniel Blain was director of the Department of Mental Hygiene of the State of California from 1957 to 1963. Capitalizing on work done previously, his influence on shaping the structure and implementation of the Short-Doyle bill which became effective in 1957, was particularly influential in making California a leader in the mental health field. Dr. Blain's remarks, coupled with those of California State Assemblyman Frank Lanterman† offer a continuity that could only be obtained from two such individuals so personally and directly involved in the developing community mental health implementation in California.

THE SHORTEST BOOK review that has come to my attention is the statement of what the book, *Sexual Life of Women*, was all about. It had followed, *The Sexual Life of Men*, these being pub-

---

* Remarks delivered at Calabasas Hospital and Health Service: Neuro-Psychiatric and Health Services, Inc., Calabasas, California, February 12, 1972.

† Co-author of the Lanterman-Petris-Short Act, 1969.

lished in the early 1930's. A friend of mine commented, "Well, all it said was, 'Women are like men, except, here and there, and now and then.'"

With due apologies to Virginia Slims, let me summarize the amazing twenty-five years of U.S. Psychiatry since World War II in seven words: "We have come a long way, Baby."

In the postwar period, we have a segment of time, which because of the great variety and strength of its forward movements, will always be remembered in my mind as the *Magic Years of U.S. Psychiatry*.[1] This was accomplished in a world in which medicine, science and society were undergoing equally dramatic and important changes, perhaps the most concentrated and exciting in the entire history of the world. We would see the development of atomic energy, following the bomb, the landing on the moon, satellite communication by television and radio, major advances in physics, engineering, new emphases on social and behavioral sciences, extreme developments of technology with computerized knowledge, expansion of communication in all media leading to informational overload, the breaking of the sound barrier, and such speedy travel as to interfere with the normal rhythm of human physiology. With instant communication, these changes have affected all parts of the world at a speed difficult for human adaptation.

Of Science in general, I quote from Gerald Holton, in 1961:

> Of all the scientists and research workers that have existed since the beginning of time, 90 percent are alive today. The other 10 percent have their niches in the Gallery of Time which stretches back to the thinking men who mastered fire, perhaps 100,000 years ago. This is another way of saying that the bulk of recognizable and measurable achievements of science belong to the past fifty and, preponderantly, to the past twenty-five years. In a single generation the Atomic Age has merged into the Space Age and is moving rapidly into the Nucleic Acid Age. Man has unlocked the secret of matter and released it as nuclear energy. He has burst the gravitational fences of the earth, and in the study of molecular biology is probing the secrets of life itself with implications as great as, or greater than either the atom or space. By jet and rocket, he has diminished distance and miniaturized the planet. By radio astronomy he is reaching out to the limits of the universe and recording

the broadcast signals of cosmic events of thousands of millions of years ago.[2]

In medicine, we have seen great advances such as, for example, the expansion of the antibiotics and DDT; improvements in cancer therapy; the development of the tuberculosis, cancer and heart crusades; the broadened perspective of the American Public Health Association to "Public Health and the Nation's Health"; the expansion of the tuberculosis movement to include all chest conditions; and the March of Dimes for poliomyelitis to include birth injuries. I am a product of the amazing advances in surgery, having two four-hour operations inside the chest within nine months. The amazing advances in anesthesiology must have been most helpful to permit the surgeon to go to open heart surgery, organ transplants and the suturing of blood vessels and nerve trunks. We have seen internal medicine moving toward the primary physician to be joined by pediatrics, public health and psychiatry. The practice of pediatrics, limited because of the antibiotics, permitted these specialists to give more time to the emotional problems of both children and parents, and to move into the field of retardation. Psychosomatic medicine has moved rapidly ahead, with two journals devoted to it.

It is impossible to cover adequately, even though briefly, changes in the society and political life around the world. We have seen the United States emerge as world leader with untold wealth, military power and political prestige, and the responsibilities which these have brought. All this while whole colonial empires have been transformed into independent republics.

In this atmosphere of proliferation and advancement, psychiatry has moved ahead as never before.

What were the antecedents of this phenomenal growth? Perhaps a suitable introduction to where we are now would be to touch lightly on several items from my own experience. Going back to 1929, the year of my medical school graduation, all I can remember of psychiatry is that there was nothing for the medical student until his senior year. Then, we were given a series of six lectures on mental disease and neuropathology, each accompanied by a visit to the nearby state hospital where we were shown a classical museum piece of essentially deteriorated patients.

Now, psychiatry is scheduled for all four years, frequently introducing the whole patient for the first time to new medical students. I recall the American Board of Psychiatry and Neurology was formed in 1934, the fifth of what are now nineteen specialty boards. About the middle of that decade the first specific treatment for a major mental illness was introduced; the insulin shock process. This was followed quickly and briefly by Metrazol®, and then electro-convulsive therapy, still in use. Residency training in psychiatry started about the time of the American boards. I did not take a residency, continuing on in my apprenticeship type of exposure, with supervision by older psychiatrists. In the late 1930's before the war, the Veterans Administration and state hospitals came to my attention in an unfavorable light, for opportunities there were meager. Commonwealth fellowships in mental hygience were offered at $1,800 a year.

Contrary to the experience of mental hospitals, the Marine Hospitals of the U.S. Public Health Service were in critical manpower shortages (my wife was a patient there) and patient care fell to a low ebb. But because of their fine public relations, they escaped entirely the condemnation of the V.A.[3] and state hospitals[4] at the end of the war period. State hospitals were getting more and more overcrowded. Subject to a study in 1937 by the Public Health Service, the APA, and the National Committee on Mental Hygiene, they appeared in a dismal condition. Only the development of psychopathic hospitals, begun in 1902 in Michigan, offered a faint scientific light on the potentials of state government.[5] During the war in 1943, state hospitals of New York were seriously condemned by the Moreland Commission. At the same time, private practice was more and more popular, and doctors were refusing to join public institutions.

Psychoanalysis was moving ahead rapidly in popular esteem, and I, myself, in 1933 voiced the belief that to be qualified in psychoanalysis appeared to be more important than to be certified by the American Board of Psychiatry and Neurology. However, I took the board exams in 1937, and luckily, passed, helped by a leading question concerning the Red Nucleus, when only about 40 percent were making the grade on the first attempt. It was the neurology material which was so difficult. It wasn't until the two were separated into two distinct branches of medicine, and the term *neuropsychiatry* fell out of common use, that the boards eased up on their pressure on the difficult neurological section. I completed formal training in psychoanalysis in 1938.

The National Committee on Mental Hygiene had been moving ahead, with little fanfare since 1909, but with increasing influence.[6] Its leader, during World War I, Dr. Thomas Salmon, emerged as one of the leading physicians in the country.[7] But the time was not ready for psychiatry to move ahead even with that considerable war impetus. The National Committee on Mental Hygiene was primarily interested in research in schizophrenia, supported by Scottish-Rite Masonry; and in child guidance clinics, which were spoken of in terms of *preventive psychiatry*. There are no figures that ever have been brought to bear to indicate their influence. The National Committee sponsored the National Association for Psychiatric Clinics for Children, which acted as the *approving board* for all child psychiatric clinics.[8]

The general status of psychiatry was not high. It was rarely separated from medicine in medical school curricula, or in the rotating internship. Barbiturates were the main drugs used. Psychotherapy was just beginning to have a respectable core curriculum for training, primarily because of psychoanalytic training.

During World War II, the beginning of which is now thirty years behind us, there was marked depletion of all civilian psychiatric services due to the military demands, and it was natural that criticism of all governmental institutions became common talk. Their inherent weaknesses were amplified by further depletion, during the war, but some hospitals with strong programs were able to maintain them. During the war, mental disorders stuck out like a sore thumb when a million and a half persons were turned down by draft boards. Correctness of these decisions is highly questionable, since they allowed only two or three minutes per man for the psychiatric examination.

Thousands were released from military service with psychiatric disabilities. Consequently, a high percentage of all handicapped persons, emerging into veteran's status, became the responsibility of the Psychiatry, Neurology and Psychology Division of the V.A. On the other hand, military services distinguished themselves in the handling of combat fatigue, the syndrome which succeeded the term *shellshock* of WWI. The near absence of major hysteria in WWII was in great contrast with the previous war. Physicians returned with personal experience with emotional problems of the soldiers, and showed great interest in psychiatry.

Our field emerged from the war with some of the major leaders in the medical world. For example, in the Offices of the Surgeon General of the different services, there were Brig. Gen. William C. Menninger, Admiral Francis Braceland, and Asst. Surgeon General of the PHS, Robert H. Felix—all distinguished gentlemen. The head of the merchant marine program was selected to head the postwar V.A. psychiatric program.

Conscientious objectors during the war were not excused, but were placed in what was known as Civilian Public Service, or CPS.[9] Among the 12,000 of these were some 3,000 assigned to fifty-seven different state hospitals; many of these were from the Society of Friends, or Quakers, and there were some 1,500 from the Mennonite Church. It was these CPS people who organized, after the war, the Mental Health Foundation which joined with the National Committee of Mental Hygiene in the National Association for Mental Health; their purpose to put their shoulders behind the effort to improve the lot of mentally ill patients in state hospitals.

During the war, a program was carried out for merchant seamen who had broken down following torpedoing by German submarines, causing thousands to become incapacitated.[10] This program was carried out during the war in six small psychiatric institutions which were called *rest centers*. There, after a mandatory stay of three weeks, a very strong total push program was developed, with a maximum of social uplift in confidence-restoring techniques, with adequate individual and group psychotherapy.

Ten thousand sailors used this program on a voluntary basis, ninety percent of whom returned to sea. The slang expression *combat fatigue* in the army and *convoy fatigue*, as the seamen called it, were actually the first of the mental disorders listed in the Army nomenclature, known as *transient situational reaction*.[11]

In his book, published in 1948, *Psychiatry and a Troubled World: Yesterday's War and Today's Challenge*, General Menninger was *prophetic* in calling upon his colleagues to put psychiatry into a public policy role as the only branch of medicine interested in the whole person. He felt that we should integrate Medicine into public problems, and he mentioned specifically race relations, unemployment, war, housing shortages, even foreign policy. Menninger was almost *evangelistic* for the profession and its teaching, as shown in the title and introduction of the book.[12]

So at war's end, beginning in the summer of 1945, and pushed by the demand for psychiatric services for returning veterans, great and rapid movement occurred in every aspect of psychiatry, both as a science and as a profession, and in psychiatry's social partners; mental health and mental retardation. There was advancement of psychiatric knowledge expanded by research, demonstrated particularly in treatment techniques which now are moving in every possible area of experimentation. Increased numbers became involved in psychiatric education which was broadened in content through three national congresses on education in psychiatry and accompanied by the development of greater manpower resources in associated professional persons and the use of persons less trained. Organizational advances took place in community and administrative psychiatry with the development of a new framework for all psychiatric operations, especially in the nonhospital programs; there was also extraordinary participation by general hospitals.

There were new methods of administration, particularly the geographic unit system. There were advances in architecture for general and mental institutions and in the amounts of money available from multiple sources. There were back-up social services for people's needs in addition to the direct therapy they were receiving. Relations with the law and the courts and with ministers of religion and the churches improved.[13] But perhaps most importantly of all was the unexpected success in the creation of better understanding by the public and increased support given to mental health legislation and appropriations.

These movements in psychiatry have worked together to place psychiatrists at a distance from other physicians, and separated from medicine. At the same time, as an independent specialty, it has gained in respect and stature. Psychiatry has moved faster toward public service and social needs. It has reduced the unoccupied space between the isolated efforts of state hospitals and the offices of private practitioners.

There is considerable improvement in the distribution of psychiatrists.[14] The total number has increased from 3,000 in 1948 to about 25,000 in 1971; and these are moving out of the metropolitan areas into suburbs, and more and more frequently into small rural centers of population. The utilization of their time has also changed. Whereas many psychiatrists were previously involved 100 percent of their time in private practice, now nearly all give one-fourth to one-third of their time in consultation, teaching and part-time salaried positions in public services. Salaried psychiatrists, on the other hand, traditionally working full-time in state institutions and in private hospitals, are more and more giving some of their time to private practice, to teaching and research and consultation away from and out of the hours of their regular salaried position.

In my mind, the chief development of psychiatry in these years, has been the quiet evolutionary movement toward increased emphasis on environmental aspects of patients' needs, and a new form of framework; community psychiatry.[15] In the early influence of psychoanalysis great progress was made in understanding intrapsychic phenomena. Now, without diminishing the importance of the intrapsychic area, the world around the patient is brought into focus at an increasing level of importance, so that the two are approaching equal emphasis. These developments, particularly increased improvements in therapy, have led to a gradual change in the framework in which we have been able to make our technical services available.

We have moved into a system of delivery of mental health services which now combine all varieties of previously isolated and separate programs. These now can be listed as *the slimmed down novalescent state hospital;* the burgeoning world of private psychiatric hospitals, private practicing psychiatrists, groups of physicians and psychiatrists, and treatment outside of hospitals near the patients, with a horde of associated personnel in psychology, social work, and nursing service with varying degrees of training and skill working with them. All of this is enlightened by improvements in administration and organization which have brought mental facilities into the computer age.

All of these are included in a type of systematic relatedness, or social organization known as *comprehensive community mental health and retardation centers.* Ideally, such centers operate a beltline of services in which the state hospital is only a small, temporary station. The keynote of these centers is the *acceptance of responsibility for a designated geographical area, and I believe it is this responsibility for a given population,* which is the essence of what some people claim is a new specialty in psychiatry—community psychiatry.

However, let us remember that the idea of the importance of the environment, and the interaction between the patient and the people and physical conditions around him, is nothing new. Attention to these interpersonal and environmental relationships of our patients has been going on for years. Even psychoanalysis, condemned by many for concentrating on the intrapersonal structure of the personality, and overemphasizing the past, actually deals with the patient's reaction to his environment in every single session. This system of treatment is misunderstood these days. The essence of the analytic process is that a procedure has been developed which permits the least amount of interference with the thinking and emotional reactions of the patient in treatment, particularly his reactions to what the analyst is doing, or showing in his movements and his face; and avoidance of fatigue and bodily sensations and hence; the couch. The whole process is so organized that the natural resistance to bringing out unconscious painful and anxiety-ridden material will be kept as low as possible; all to the end that the patient is assisted in continuing treatment rather than running away.

It is now obvious that this technique is applicable to perhaps only 5 percent of patients,[16] but where the fundamental change of personality is necessary, all other treatment having failed, I firmly believe that nothing else can take its place. It is primarily useful in deep and serious neuroses which can be as devastatingly crippling to a patient and his family as any psychosis or personality disorder. I say a small percentage should be treated this way, but the Freudian technique will continue to be useful for research purposes, and particularly for the general principles and further knowledge of the psyche, which again, I believe, must continue to dominate our total concept of mental health and human personality.

The handling of patients outside of large isolated state institutions, and treating them near their homes, is of course facilitated by enormous increase and improvements in treatment techniques. All of these factors have assisted in the placing of the person close to the appropriate treatment process, combined operationally into a new psychiatric delivery system.

I believe that what we have been doing all these years has been generally good, despite much of today's criticism, where we were able to apply the knowledge which we have had. Now we have added refinements and a new dimension. In my opinion, all good psychiatry in the future will include the *community concept*. Therefore, I see no merit in the idea that community psychiatry may develop into another subspecialty of psychiatry as a whole. The same broad approaches which assist in the development of this aspect of our work, are equally needed and demanded in hospital work, private practice, in industrial and other forms of psychiatric practice.

I think we can claim a real system of delivery of mental health and retardation services which provide immediate and available access to 24-hour emergency stations in all centers. Given a few more months or years to perfect our system, we have something here which is available now to all classes of persons who need brief appointments, social service contacts, day services, day hospitals, scheduling of day activities, short-term brief hospitalization; and if those fail, there are still other hospitals which can accommodate them for somewhat longer periods of time, but hopefully with limits on the length of stay.

We have a system which provides what I mentioned above, a beltline of identification, diagnosis, treatment, rehabilitation, resocialization, beginning and ending at home, or a suitable substitute thereof. All of these opportunities must ideally be available for the patient somewhere near his place of residence, and they must be truly available, accessible, and acceptable to all people.

The roots of the community services idea have been planted years ago, and in the early 1950's were described as *the current new look in American psychiatry* in many publications, and also in the burgeoning ideas of many innovative persons of all types in the field of mental health and retardation. In 1952, the World Health Organization studied the concept of the *Community Mental Hospital* and issued a report in the name of the expert committee on mental health called for that purpose. In 1956, in a survey of the state of Iowa of its mental health resources, the APA Report included a chapter called, New Ideas. These included, "community mental health centers, branch hospitals, day hospitals, night hospitals, halfway houses, sheltered workshops, rehabilitation hospitals, therapeutic farms, diagnostic and screening centers, small private residential units, private psychiatric hospitals, psychiatric units in general hospitals, mental health clinics, the offices of psychiatrists and other associated persons in private practice."[17]

In 1958, the Butler Hospital of Providence, Rhode Island, became in effect an early if not the first comprehensive mental health center.[18] After closing its 160 beds in 1956 for financial reasons, and after having been studied by an APA Committee, the Butler Hospital reopened its doors with forty beds, a large day hospital operation, and rented various buildings to more than ten community agencies; all associated together on the same ground. The staff, for a time, also persuaded two out of three patients, arriving with family and baggage, to go home and return to the day hospital unit.

Three important training centers in community psychiatry have

been in operation in Berkeley, California, New York City and
Boston.

Each of the items I have mentioned in this expanding portfolio
of treatment services deserves more detailed and thoughtful discussion than is possible in a limited paper. These ideas have been
exemplified in a number of operations, programs, movements,
developments, and the like. Let me name some of these:

1. Psychiatry in the Veterans Administration. The V.A. program has had 60,000 in-patient beds, and some 400,000 contacts
in out-patient services, screening examinations, etc. a year.
Sparked by overwhelming criticism and demands, the V.A. was to
have the first opportunity to present new ideas into operation. It
made important contributions in organization and administration, including architecture and the inclusion of psychiatric
services in all general medical and surgical hospitals. Also new
formulas for raising standards of treatment[19] and the creation of a
psychiatric residency program and a clinical psychology Ph.D.
program through association with medical schools and universities; the largest in the world, and the invention of the Deans
Committee.

2. The second major cluster of operations bring together the
amazing contributions which followed the organization, expansion and development of some forty-five national professional organizations devoted to our field, many founded after World War
II. The first of these, chronologically at least, was the rebellion
of the American Psychiatric Association which took place in
May 1946. I am proud to state that this organization, the oldest
national medical organization in the United States, has not only
been the leader for improvements of psychiatric profession and
services from within, but as an organization has repeatedly revised its efforts to meet the challenge: "Is the APA so organized
and operated as to meet the changing needs and demands for
psychiatric services in the U.S.A.?"[20]

3. In two months after the APA meeting, there occurred the
second significant event in the federal government, the Enabling
Act which was to produce three years later the National Institute
of Mental Health and the beginning of the ongoing program
of the Social Security Agency, now the Department of Health,

Education and Welfare. This was the national Mental Health Act of July 3, 1946.[21] Contrary to the Veterans Administration program, this federal agency has been concerned only in a very minimal way with operating clinical services. Its major function has been the planning, and to some degree, the regulation of programs which it financed through direct categorical appropriations from the Congress.

The program consisted at first (1) of the training of four categories of graduate education: psychiatrists, clinical psychologists, psychiatric social workers, and psychiatric nurses; (2) research in mental health; and (3) the promotion of community services. One bow was made to the needs of patients in state mental hospitals through grants known as Hospital Improvement Programs (HIP). They assisted in preparing patients to leave the hospitals. One grant was provided for each hospital for ten years. Later, other categories and activities were added. The NIMH has exceeded all other institutes of health in size, broad scope of activities, and its 600 million dollar budget (1971).

4. The state hospital system: two words cover its 25-year record—*scandal* and *recovery*. These hospitals grew in population each year until about 1955, when NIMH was proud to announce in 1956 for the first time a reduction in the ranks of the overcrowded institutions. In the fifteen years since, the reduction in state hospital population has gone from 550,000 to 300,000. These drops are largely credited to pharmacological products but some of us believe that equal importance must be attributed to the increases in activity programs and other treatments and in followup services into the community, which has reduced the numbers of patients coming back.

This was most dramatically shown in California which has used about half the amount of ataractic drugs per one hundred patients as compared to the rest of the nation; has had an outstanding program of activities and organized social work followup, and the fastest drop of state hospital population in the nation. In general, one must credit the cooperation of Governors, Governors' conferences, The Council of State Government, state legislators and citizens' groups, with an appreciable amount of professional leadership in the APA district branch societies and mental health societies. The increased availability of local services in the last two years has been a strong determinant in further reduction of hospital census. These hospitals still have a long way to go and a new function to perform.

5. The total group of activities designated as the private sector of American psychiatry comes next.[22] These include private practicing professionals, private hospitals, clinics, voluntary hospitals, with and without psychiatric units, and also the large number of welfare agencies, foundations, industrial health services, labor-contracted benefits, churches, schools, and contributions of higher education operating on a private basis. These add up to far greater persons and services and production than the government institutions already mentioned. They include also the citizens' movements, which will be described next. The private sector, of course, really includes the contributions of the 200 million persons in the country. Even those who work for the government still have 128 hours a week to tend to their own private business and to assume responsibilities of other citizens in any area in which they are concerned.

Related to the private sector are the relations between public and private psychiatric services. In most of our activities today, it is hard to find any operation which is entirely private, or entirely governmental. The importance of both contributors is increasing regularly as time goes on. In general, the federal government provides tax monies for operations in which the authorities are governmental employees, but federal tax money also subsidizes privately managed concerns to some degree. These include: assistance in education, particularly special education; health programs under private management, and almost all aspects of growth and development particularly institutions that help handicapped persons, the poor and the aged of every type. Some of these opportunities for help in grants, projects, and research are limited as far as institutions go to nonprofit organizations. But individuals can apply for various kinds of help regardless of their connections, including research grants and subsidies for worthwhile projects.

Neither government nor private agencies go all the way in terms of assuming responsibility. For example, state hospitals and clinics are operated on state tax money, but the family and the patient's estate are called upon to contribute when they can. This amounted to an average of 10 percent of the budget of the Department of Mental Hygiene when I was there in 1959 to 1963. In my opinion, any institutions who are close enough to share their resources and ideas and their professional competence and advice should have every encouragement to work together and cooperate in terms of resources and their needs.

One of the great nongovernmental agencies was the lobbying organization known as the National Committee Against Mental Illness, for which Mrs. Mary Lasker and Mr. Mike Gorman operated the greatest influential agent towards securing federal legislation and appropriations for Mental Health and Retardation until the latter was separated from Mental Health, and carried on under its own pressure system.[23]

6. The next of these *agents of change* are the citizens' movements. It is not generally recognized that these are a very distinct American type of operation, early adopted with great potency by our Canadian friends. These are the mental health movement, led primarily by the National Association of Mental Health, formed in 1949 from earlier roots,[24] and the retardation movement, led primarily by the National Association for Retarded Children, formed in 1950.[25] These are true citizens' movements, made up of a cross section of all peoples.

Their major functions, I believe, are public education; the development of interest and support for highly-recommended programs for the mentally ill and retarded, and watch dogs of the establishment and consumer. These two associations, and their state and local branches, are chiefly responsible for great changes in the public's understanding and the strong support which we have received. They are well organized, and have produced a most forceful kind of influence, emanating from a large number of voters to which our representatives in government pay due attention. There are also occasional programs for mental health and retardation, put on by a number of important groups; for example, the Junior Chamber of Commerce, the League of Women Voters, the Association of University Women, religious groups, veterans associations, local groups all over the country, and others.

7. The last group, which I will discuss only briefly, is composed of international psychiatric and related organizations which have sprung up during this period of time. The APA, founded in 1844, has itself been multinational since 1945, when Canada was invited to join. And further, in 1952, Mexico, Central America and the Carribean were brought into its regular membership. Worldwide associations began in June 1948, when the First Assembly of the World Health Organization (WHO) met in Geneva. In July 1948 the First Assembly of the World Federation of Mental Health met. This worldwide group in London received the shock, which all of us felt, delivered by the WHO the month before. We were brought face to face with a serious weakness. Mental health was refused a first priority in its oncoming program; whereas tuberculosis, venereal disease, malaria, sanitation, and other programs qualified. We failed because we did not meet two of the three adopted criteria. We met the first, which was a universal need for psychiatric services. We failed the second that there must be available mass techniques for primary prevention and for treatment. And we failed the third, because techniques that were available must be economical in terms of money, manpower and time. We still have not met those criteria.

The World Psychiatric Association was formed after several independent world congresses in Montreal, in 1961. The President and the first vice-president for this first period of time, were Dr. D. Ewen Cameron and Dr. Francis Braceland, both of the United States, though Cameron was chairman in McGill at the time.

Of greatest interest, perhaps to us, was the InterAmerican Council of Psychiatric Associations, formed in 1965. This includes all the countries of the Western hemisphere. It is distinctly an American program for all the Americas. Its objectives include exchanges of information, ideas, studies of common problems, mutual assistance in research, training, and the holding of conferences. For example, an important hemispheric conference entitled, *Mental Health of the Americas* was held in San Antonio,

Texas in 1968, after three years of intensive and highly successful preparation.[26] A similar one is planned for 1973, on *Child Psychiatry in the Americas* to be held in San Juan, Puerto Rico. There are also international associations in psychoanalysis, child psychiatry, social psychiatry, group psychotherapy, neurology, retardation, sociology, psychology, and others. The World Medical Association was formed in this period, as were international groups in almost all the specialties of medicine.

Each of these seven topics deserves an entire book for adequate coverage. Together they give us pretty much the operations and organizations in which the great forward movements and specialized efforts in mental health and retardation have occurred. There remain several dramatic occurrences, which to some degree illustrate the points that I have raised. Following that, I would like to name a few of our successes, a few of our weaknesses, and indicate briefly the directions to which our current situations and thinking seem to point.

The first of these dramatic events is what I like to call *Appel's Appeal.* In October 1953, Kenneth E. Appel, president of the APA, made an appeal to the nation at the Mental Health Institute in Little Rock, Arkansas.[27] He spoke of the failure of the hospital system. He called for greater professional leadership, particularly among American psychiatrists, who he felt had the greatest responsibility. He demanded a national study as far-reaching as the Flexner Report for medical schools in 1909. The timing was right, the voice was strong, the response was immediate. The nation and the Congress and the Administration were ready. Thirty-six organizations formed a Joint Commission on Mental Illness and Health, of which Dr. Appel became president. The Congress unanimously passed the Mental Health Act of 1955, signed immediately by President Eisenhower. This provided, in a new precedent, one and one-fourth million dollars to be matched in part by private funds, the work to be done by a private organization on contract with the National Institute of Mental Health. The Joint Commission was chosen as the agent. The report was completed, and given to President Kennedy in 1961. It consisted of a summation volume called, *Action on Mental*

Health. It was accompanied by arrangements for special volumes on ten major topics, to be written by selected individuals. These, with one or two exceptions, were published by Basic Books.

The result was, under Kennedy's sponsorship, appropriations in 1961 for funds to every state to conduct a large-scale, two-year study of needs, trends and resources in mental health. (Mental retardation was not included because it was in the process of separation from the NIMH.) Congress provided forty-one million dollars for this, of which California and New York received some $450,000; and Pennsylvania, one of the large states, $400,000. Compare this with the $5,000 to $20,000 the APA used to make mental health surveys in some fifteen states in the decade before, and to break new ground in using public hearings in all major centers to create a ground swell to mental health. On February 5, 1963, the President gave the first speech from the White House on a health subject.[28] It was entitled "Mental Health and Retardation." He called for a *bold, new approach.* Congress passed the Comprehensive Mental Health Construction Act in 1963, calling for equal matching money from some other source; and the following year, 1964, provided federal monies to pay for staffing for four years, diminishing each year. Thus was created the federal support and demand for mental health centers, comprehensive in scope, each to provide all necessary mental health care for a total population in catchment areas of 75 to 200,000 people. Some 2,000 of these throughout the nation have been planned.

The second dramatic event was in January 1958 when the movement toward community-based programs was in the air and when the Commissioner of Mental Health of the Province of Ontario, Canada at the Mental Hospital Institute in Toronto, reported that his doctors, although they feared the loss of their jobs in the apparent early demolition of state hospitals, nevertheless felt that as physicians they must not let anything stand in the way of what mentally ill patients needed. Therefore, they presented and recommended for action the following formula, which I like to call *McNeel's Ideal.*[29] This was based on Canada's Mental Health Study, and was presented on this occasion by Ontario mental hospital doctors. It went as follows: Adequate treatment must be available (accessible, acceptable): (1) as early as possible; (2) as continuously as possible; (3) with as little dislocation as possible, and (4) with as much social restoration as possible. This did in fact anticipate President Kennedy's *bold, new approach* for it meant an appreciable shift in timing, location, use of resources and follow-through to adequate social adjustment.

A third dramatic event occurred in 1954, when New York passed the first state-county mental health law, providing state financing to county programs.[30] This occurred shortly after the Department of Mental Hygiene, at the request of Governor Dewey, was challenged by a committee investigating crimes perpetuated by former mental hospital patients. The challenge was to spend as much money outside of state hospitals as was spent inside. California followed in 1957 with the Short-Doyle Law, and now has gone much further in turning over authority and responsibility to the counties in the 1969 Lanterman-Petris-Short Law.[31] A number of states followed, including New Jersey; in 1965 Michigan; in 1966 Pennsylvania, and many since.

The Pennsylvania Mental Health Code is a good example of what the states were doing, and also the legislation that is necessary in all states to meet the demand in matching monies, and in state financing to meet the opportunities presented by the federal government, and to produce what is now in effect, ahead of all other branches of medicine, a potentially satisfactory delivery system for mental health and retardation services.

The state provides 90 percent of the county program, and in Pennsylvania, it is mandated in every county within one year of the passage of the Law. This provides immediate access to twenty-four-hour emergency service for all people of all ages in each catchment area, which will, hopefully, cover the entire state, and the nation. A successful example of this program occurs in the city of Philadelphia, with two million people and one mental hospital devoted entirely to the city. It has appreciable psychiatric resources. Its population is divided into eleven catchment areas, of which nine are operative. These are under a variety of sponsorships, such as general hospitals, private psychiatric hospitals, medical schools, and consumer associations, and the

like. Coverage, which is moving rapidly toward the entire city, is
made up of these Centers, all using the Philadelphia State Hospital, known as "Byberry" as a back-up resource.

Byberry, recently, was one of the largest, most overcrowded
and poorly-administered hospitals in the nation. The admission
rate has now been cut from 2,200 in 1966 to approximately 800
in 1970. Patients returning from the community to the hospital,
are about one-third as many as were coming back previously, but,
of course, not the same patients who left the hospital in any given
period of time. The hospital has shrunk from 6,100 to 2,100 in
five years, and is moving down to only 1,000. It acts as a station on
the beltline of psychiatric care that any patient may use, starting
at his own home, and finally, hopefully, ending up at his own
home, with none of the way stations such as the old-time mental
hospital conceived as the end of the line. Catchment areas which
do not have complete resources, can, by contract, utilize beds or
services in other areas. A number of important problems exist but
all of these have potentials for being handled.

The fourth dramatic occurrence was the invention of the
Deans' Committee and its adoption by the authorities of the Veterans Administration in 1945, probably the greatest single shot
in the arm to the relief of medical manpower that has ever occurred.[32] Along with the rest of the medical services, the forty
hospitals which are predominantly psychiatric, have contracted,
with a few exceptions, with deans of medical schools to supervise
residency training in psychiatry and neurology. This included also
supervision of treatment activities, and maintaining them at
a high standard by the medical school authorities. Within three
months of the passage of Public Law 293, 77th Congress, January
3, 1946, the Psychiatry and Neurology Division reported 100 psychiatric residents in training, half of whom were at the Menninger
School of Psychiatry, located at Topeka Veterans Hospital, Kansas, under the aegis of the Menninger Foundation.

Within a year and a half, there were 500 psychiatrists in training in 30 of the hospitals; and within the same period of time, 500
candidates for Ph.D.'s in psychology, training under the same general Deans Committee plan. Each of these has graduated over 3,000
students in the last 25 years. The essence of the Deans Committee

idea was a verbal agreement to participate on the part of the medical school with assignment of staff, and of the V.A. to furnish opportunities for placing on the payroll members of the faculty on whole or part-time to carry out the residency training program. This produced a combined program in which there was no exchange of money between the two organizations, and no documents were officially signed. This has been a miracle in dealings between government and private agencies.

The fifth dramatic occurrence was the battle over Medicare, finalized in 1965. There has been a struggle since 1935, when the first Social Security legislation passed by the Congress provided many benefits, but included one ominous statement, "These benefits shall not be available to those who have ever been in a mental hospital, or have a diagnosis of psychosis." I understand this was done on the doubtful basis that such benefits were already rendered by the state. The 1952 Amendment to give benefits to those with complete and total disability contained the same statement. The Murray-Wagner-Dingle Bill, providing for a system of medical care, and revised in the 1940's, contained the same statement.

The Republican version of this attempt to revise the health delivery system, known as the Kerr Bill, 1958, contained the same monotonous denial to mental patients; and finally the Medicare Bill which was in Congress several years, again stuck to the old line. Protests were made again and again, but always met with the response, "It is too expensive and the states are doing it." The matter was brought before the governors, by Governor Edmund G. "Pat" Brown of California in 1959, and in subsequent Governors' Conferences. There were direct discussions with Mr. Wilbur Cohen, Deputy Secretary of HEW for legislation. I was one of the proponents for this fight. It got so he recognized me, and would shout across the meeting room, "Keep going, Blain, you'll get what you want!"

In 1962, Mr. Cohen informed me of the report of the President's Committee on Social Welfare, appointed by President Eisenhower, which had reported in 1961, and suggested revising the Social Security Laws to include mental patients. It recommended certain criteria be met: (1) there would be no duplication of services already rendered by the state; (2) new services would be provided by new federal money; and (3) cost estimates be provided which showed the extra cost would not be excessive. Efforts were then made to obtain such cost estimates.

In 1965, it was obvious that Johnson had the votes, and the Medicare Bill would be passed. Efforts were redoubled. Without entering the fight over Medicare or no Medicare, the position was taken that if such benefits were to be given to the majority of elderly people of the country, mental patients should not be *included out*. The NIMH failed to come forth with cost estimates. Meetings were held with HEW representatives and some members of Congress. Finally, at the request of the APA President, the National Association of Private Mental Hospitals appointed Dr. Robert Gibson in January, 1965 to represent them, and he and I came up with some estimates from the records of states and private hospitals, which indicated the extra cost would be lower than had been believed in the past, and were within reason.

Several days before the Bill came to a vote, I saw Mr. Lawrence O'Brien in the White House. He was closest to the Johnson Administration. I told him that the public would not stand for the elimination of the mentally ill poor in mental hospitals from these supposedly magnificent benefits, and he expressed surprise that the bill was worded in this way. The next day, the White House, through Mr. Wilbur Cohen, announced it had withdrawn its opposition to the inclusion of mental patients. A number of Congressmen spoke out immediately, including Senator McCarthy and Senator Ribicoff. A compromise was made for mental patients in state hospitals, who were given a partial set of benefits, and not as liberal as for the rest of the nation, but an opening wedge had been achieved.

A sequel to this really great victory is contained in the ten or more current proposals for national health insurance in 1970.[33] Only one of these contains very limited benefits for mental patients in general hospitals and out-patient services. But none will include all of the patients who were now in the state hospital system. The argument is that the extra cost would be so great that the people would not favor the bill, and legislation would be lost. Better a compromise, even though they be excluded. The decisions were political, and not based on the needs of people. "Let them eat cake."

The next dramatic occurrences which I want to mention in this magnificent period of time occurred one day in September, 1966. I was sitting at lunch at a Committee Meeting on Personal Health Services of the National Commission on Community Health Services, in Philadelphia. This was the subcommittee under Dr. I. V. Ravdin, famed surgeon of the University of Pennsylvania. I found myself sitting next to Dr. Melvin Glasser, a political scientist who had been involved in public service, and had been executive director of the White House Conference on "Children and Youth" in 1950, where I had known him.

I said, "Mel, what are you doing now?" I knew he had been the vice president of Brandeis University in Massachusetts.

He said, "I've just moved to the Social Security Division of the United Automobile Workers in Detroit."

I said, "I believe that your group is in a position to do something we've been needing a long time. We must have some private agency to make a major demand for the extension of health insurance into the field of mental illness, equal to the coverage of other fields of health, but extended over into the doctor's office, out-patient clinic, and other nonhospital services."

He replied, "We've been thinking of doing something like that. Do you think that the questions which have kept this from occurring in the past can really be answered?"

I said, "Yes, I have no doubt about it."

Two weeks later, Dr. Glasser brought his major assistant from Detroit to my office in Philadelphia. He went into the difficulties which were most often recounted, such as: Can mental illness be defined? Can one predict the length of care? Can we measure in any reasonable way improvement and recovery? Is treatment always indefinite and without end? Will it break the system financially?

Dr. Glasser then checked my opinions with other leaders and apparently found no appreciable differences. He came to Philadelphia again for further discussions. His union included in their negotiations, as side benefits, demands for psychiatric health insurance in addition to the general hospital coverage which had already been provided, to include day hospital, doctor's office, mental hygiene clinics, etc., with one important provision, that the first five visits would be without charge, to overcome initial hesitation. These were put into the bargaining discussions with General Motors, Chrysler, Ford and American Motors. The APA appointed a Committee which assisted the union in their planning. I personally sat in at a meeting with Ford to answer questions on both sides. These benefits were granted and the first breakthrough of out-patient coverage for any medical group were granted to mental patients. The first few years have already demonstrated that the demand was not excessive. Enough psychiatric help was available to cover the extra demand. The program was feasible. The same benefits have since been secured by the steel industry and are spreading to other industries.[34]

One more dramatic event occurs to me worthy of mention. While conducting a public hearing in Wilkes-Barre, Pennsylvania in 1955 in the APA Mental Health Survey of Pennsylvania, a General Family Service Agency reported serving some 500 families in which although in no case the chief complaint, there were obvious emotional problems in some eighty percent of the families. A six-months' check-up showed that after providing general relief from the disturbing social situation, only about ten percent needed psychiatric consultation, and two percent of the families had one member enter a mental hospital.

But there were some 500 other families requesting assistance which could not be given. Information obtained, however, indicated that a high percentage of these families also had important emotional problems, and a six months' check later on showed that these unserved families showed demoralization and frequent break-up of the family. Nearly all needed specific psychiatric help, and an appreciable number required mental hospitalization. The APA survey team pondered on such questions as, "What happens to these people under stress which ended in their becoming psychiatric casualties? And what failed to happen to people which might have prevented them from moving so far in this direction?"

These queries resulted in dividing all people into what we call *Zonal Classification of People*.[35] These zones were (1) the unborn, until the time of delivery; (2) those born essentially normal, and remaining so until unusual stress called for special services not provided for all healthy people; (3) the zone of special need, those who had moved from Zone 1 and 2 into the group needing special health or social assistance, but not yet psychiatric cases; and (4) the zone of mental disorder, those who were born with defect or later developed diagnosable mental disorders or defects and were transferred from Zone 1, 2, or 3. Zone 1, 2, and 3 are areas where primary prevention and positive mental health programs could be organized. Each zone has with it a listing of the necessary services which should be available, and could be a check list.

This whole plan was introduced as a working plan for guidance in developing various forms of assistance, and checking the population to evaluate the load. It is important to note that only in Zone 4 would there be fully-employed, trained mental health personnel. Competent mental health persons would be useful as consultants to people working in Zones 1, 2, and 3 for guidance and advice. This is offered also as a practical *unassembled* program in both positive mental health and primary prevention. Prevention in this instance is essentially aimed at assisting people who have intolerable stress from developing anxiety which is beyond their capacity to handle as individuals, particularly to intervene before a psychiatric condition was developed. Looking back, this apparently anticipates the current demand to include total population.

So we come to the late 1960's, with great expansion, increased manpower, strong departments of psychiatry in virtually every medical school, with many of the best senior students going into psychiatry, strong financial backing in the Congress, up and down support in the states depending on individual governors, but consistently strong public support, which has kept the extremists from drastically cutting programs, both in the Congress and in the various states. There has been increased training in nonprofessional areas, the relief of pressure on hospitalization, and movement toward less expensive treatment for ambulatory patients who compose, after all, the great majority of mental patients. And there has been created, and is in operation, a system of delivery of mental health services which includes easy access and total coverage, a generally encouraging picture over the whole range of psychiatric treatment services.

CHALLENGES

Then appeared challenges to our complacency. The world around us emitted danger signals. An early warning came from an editorial in the *Journal of the Explorers Club*, ordinarily devoted to physical and geographical matters:

> The startling and frightening fact is the rate at which man's technology creates fear—and new problems which he cannot solve. Medicine and public health are doubling human populations every few years, and soon we won't know where the food is coming from. The need for more room on earth increases tensions between peoples, and we don't know how to relieve them short of war. Nuclear science has made the bomb—an instrument of possible total death—and we don't know how to keep it out of the hands of irresponsibles. We live in a world so lacking in the understanding of social and human problems that gentle solutions are not remotely in sight. So we spend much of our energies, and use a large part of our miraculous technological skills, making bombs and navies and air forces that could one day end it all for us.[36]

We were alerted to overpopulation, the information overload, urban build-up with rural depletion, megalopolis complicated by "death of the cities," pollution of water, air and food in the sea. There were serious prophecies of possible extinction of life on this earth. Real advances have been followed by demands for instant health, instant equality and opportunity, instant elimination of poverty, and an expanding list of *rights* with little talk of *responsibility*.

All of this was complicated by general demoralization of adults and dishonesty in people at every level, failure of family life and guidance to the young, many of whom have lost their confidence in authority and the law, and our prized democratic way of life, and they are joined by disappointed adults. The Vietnam War, and the chance of political and personal gain in this election period, appears to me to be the important catalyst of these extreme reactions. But we would be foolish not to search out whatever fundamental errors and weaknesses lie hidden behind all these criticisms.

Psychiatry as a science shares the vulnerability of science in general. Harvey Brooks, the distinguished Dean of the Division of Engineering and Applied Physics at Harvard, questions the soil in which science in the United States must grow. He distinguishes between technology in which we excel, and true science. His paper, "Can Science Survive in the Modern Age?" reflects a concern about U.S. cultural trends. He questions, "whether in fact the conditions of modern society are generating a cultural climate which is no longer hospitable to the cultivation of a *true science* and whether the absence of such a viable science, in a sense expressed by Haskins, will destroy our ability to manage and control the technology which science has helped to create, and which is essential to modern civilized life."[37]

C. P. Haskins elaborates: "Only in a cultural climate where the fundamental drives of curiosity, and of the laws of discovery for its own sake are understood and cultivated, can a true science flourish. . . . It is only when such a science becomes deeply rooted as an element of high culture that a progressively innovative technology can be maintained over long periods, fusing eventually into the close partnership with which we are familiar today."[38]

And W. D. McElroy, director of the National Science Foundation, states that creative science in the United States needs a change in emphasis:

> Science as one of man's highest and intellectual achievements has had a pervasive and protracted influence on man, his way of life and his environment. Destructive forces (of technology, etc.) can be properly focused and controlled and wisely used. . . . To accomplish these ends, there is necessitated a major effort on the part of Science and Scientists to serve all of society and all of man. . . . Hence the National Science Foundation must change its direction of effort. Formerly directed to academic science, the needs of the disciplines and individual scientists themselves, it must now also be strongly devoted to the social and ethnological needs of the nation. It must be a force directed to man and society and include the efforts of the large numbers of creative members of the scientific community. . . . Research and Training institutions must be more clearly focused and receptive to both immediate and long-term interests of man and society.[39]

This constant refrain of *man and society* is echoed in the field of medicine and psychiatry.

Man's great triumph in medicine has been directed toward

individual organs and diseases, and this branch of medicine; the clinical branches have dominated the profession. Another voice is now being strongly heard; not new, but increasingly strong, that of public health.

The art and science of medicine are under a cloud. The practice of medicine is labelled by many as *an industry*. Constant daily charges are made in the Congress and in the press against physicians in medical profession and the delivery of health services. The weakness of the public relation's component of organized medicine is amply demonstrated every day, and the physician's approach to individuals, and to specific organs and diseases is under serious attack. It is important to note that this criticism rarely states that the individual approach is detrimental, but rather that it is not available to enough persons to meet the needs of all the people. Hence, there are demands that the existing nonsystem be replaced by national schemes of health services; most frequently through a national insurance plan.

Now we have a split in medicine itself. Writing from the School of Public Health, University of Texas at Houston, Stalones makes the provocative statement: "The assumption that effective treatment of illness vastly improves community health is incorrect. Prolongation of life often adds to the total burden of illness in the community, and therapeutic successes sometimes increase the proportion of defective genes in the community genetic pool. . . . Most of the decline in disease incidence and mortality, and therefore most of the increase in average life expectancy has resulted from influences other than effects aimed at controlling specific diseases."[40]

He quoted a voice out of the past for a leading European public health official, who became a leader when the World Health Organization was founded in 1948, had stated as early as 1920, "No matter what the number of physicians may be, they will never improve people's health by individual therapy. . . . Practical medicine is important . . . but always for a small number of people only. . . . People's health is never in direct relation to the number of physicians."

Kotin, a pathologist, and Dean of Temple University School of Medicine said in 1972 in reenforcing this position, that the epidemic of the future will be caused by noxious products in the environment, not the bacteria in the body. The prime target, the patient, must move over and let the population take its place.[41]

In this welter of social crises and serious questions relating to our technology, and of science in general, and the sag in public opinion of the profession of medicine, there are weaknesses and unanswered questions in psychiatry and mental health; and there are serious criticisms from many directions. A candid look at these suggests that there are many grains of truth in these attacks on our current mode of operation. Far more is expected of us than we can deliver; this is in some degree a penalty of success, and there are indications that our notable moves in the general direction of *man and society* will probably swerve still further in these directions.

There are those who feel that in view of the great demonstrated needs of the day there is no room for optimism, and that enthusiastic proponents of our progress, of whom I am one, tend to exaggerate the progress and highlight the true and imagined errors.

Our greatest weakness is our inability to evaluate scientifically what has been accomplished. State legislators and the Congress, and the high price of medical services have called attention to the enormous amounts of money invested in psychiatric research, training and services. Actually, these programs, when compared to medicine in general, are still way below in numbers of physicians involved, the amount of research, and the per diem cost of public psychiatric care. But the fight for an appropriate share of the tax and private dollar demands on the part of public officials better justification than we have been able to make. Obstacles toward evaluating, toward obtaining baseline information, and the measurement of changes in behavior, emotions and other abstract components of personality disorders have not been overcome. Therefore, though there are good reasons why, we cannot measure specifically the results of our efforts in statistics and specific indices. We have plenty of subjective evidence but fail to please our critics.

There is a serious weakness in state services which, except for federal appropriations, furnish the largest amount of money for mental illness. This lies in the extraordinary influence of the personal attitudes toward mental health on the part of state governors. In some twenty state surveys carried out by APA in this 25-year period, the common experience has been that the governor and legislature, which requested a survey, and received the report, were subject to change shortly after the report was given. More often than not, this has involved a change of party in new elections. The result has been a delay in paying attention to the report. There has been satisfaction in noting that in most cases, a number of years later, the report has been taken down from the shelf, its contents noted, and most often recognized in on-going improvements.

Two states, during this period, have demonstrated the strengthening factor in a continuity of support. California has had 24 years of strong mental health support of its governors; four terms under Governor Warren, broken by his appointment to the Supreme Court. He was succeeded by another Republican, who continued his policies; and then eight years under Governor Edmund G. "Pat" Brown, a Democrat, who gave strong support to the Department of Mental Hygiene. This 24 years of steady growth, testing, consolidation and forward movement led to a remarkably high achievement record.

During this time, important work in public education by the Directors of Mental Hygiene and the State Mental Health Society and its branches produced an educated and supportive citizenry. The result was that this great strength and attitude was carried over in the state so that it was impossible for Governor Reagan to carry out his intention to reduce the forward movement in mental health; and he was forced to reverse himself and come up with a considerably larger budget than his predecessor, Governor Brown, had passed on to him. The state of New York, under the continued progressive leadership of Governor Nelson Rockefeller and other strong forces in the state, is another fortunate example of continuity of support. But the general picture is a change of governors every two or four years and very little consecutive support.

By the same token, consecutive leadership favorable to mental health has been demonstrated in the Congress, where Rep. John

Fogarty and Sen. Lister Hill continued as outstanding proponents of our interests. Of course, they were ably backed by citizens' pressure from many states, and by the extraordinary efforts of Mike Gorman and the Lasker Foundation. The obvious lesson is that where governors continue to change frequently, proponents of mental health must be developed in each of the several legislatures, and the same effort directed toward members of the Congress. On the federal level, the personal interests of the Chief Executive have been of less importance in our field until the personal relatedness of President John F. Kennedy to the field of retardation proved the power of such advocates in that field. It is probably true that no member of Congress or of the Presidency has failed to have in his family connection someone suffering from mental illness, but there has been no exposure of such facts.

On the federal level, we are meeting a serious threat to appropriations in two different ways: (1) with the greater demand for support of all manner of military and social needs competing for a weakening number of dollars, and of the strength of individual dollars, there is a demand for accounting and strong justification for mental health appropriations. This was most significantly demonstrated in the decision of the Executive Offices of the President to eliminate, by stages, support for training of psychiatrists, and to question carefully other items of the budget of the NIMH. Because of the strong support of a coalition of mental health agencies, and of pressure on members of Congress from the states, the decision was in fiscal 1972 reversed. Strong arguments emerged which appealed to the Congress to continue support, and the budget of the NIMH was raised to an all-time high. Nevertheless, it is probable that a similar attempt will be made again and before long.[42]

(2) The second major cloud on the federal horizon lies in the effort which has been increasing for some time in switching from categorical aid to discrete programs to appropriations for comprehensive programs. The argument is that specialized efforts, independent of and isolated from general health programs, for example, are inefficient, more costly, and contrary to public policy; and there is a great movement towards regional comprehensive health programs and a single health delivery system.

There is enough evidence to believe that the highly successful effort to subsidize mental health leading to an ever increasing power of NIMH over and above the resources given to other institutes of health, has played some part in this movement, which has been activated in the U.S. Public Health Service over the last few years, with strong efforts to separate the component parts of the NIMH and thus weaken its concentrated attack on one field of medicine. For the period of time in which mental illness was a grossly neglected part of the health efforts in the nation at all levels, it was essential that special pleas be made for this particular branch of medicine.

As its science has advanced, its technology improved, its professional leadership became equal, if not greater; and as mental health has shown the capacity to advance ahead of other specialties of medicine in the delivery of its services, and its current development of a potentially satisfactory mental health delivery system, the need for its isolated existence has diminished and it becomes more likely that as part of a comprehensive system, it could hold its own and even continue to flourish. This has been demonstrated in the program of the Department of Psychiatry, Neurology and Psychology in the Veterans Administration, because the conditions were suitable. But there is considerable evidence that the prejudice toward this branch of medicine is far from being overcome.

The threat of absorbing the federal program into the current planning for comprehensive health services looms as a questionable step as far as mental health services are concerned, though the advocates of equal status for mental health are growing stronger each year. The national insurance programs as mentioned above, are evidence of continued discrimination. Other strong advocates of categorical aid, however, still exist. These are: the Veterans Administration, heart, stroke and cancer proponents, retardation, and drug abuse. The strong demand of the people's lobby in many states, and in the Congress is still strong, and my belief is that this change away from categorical aid is still subject to considerable further study, and Congress will approach it with caution.

Special criticisms and challenges to current Mental Health activities come from many directions; from the lay public, professionals in various fields and some of our own psychiatrists, and there are grains of truth in all these criticisms.

There is questioning of our standards, nomenclature, and classifications of disorders; of the effects of white, middle-class approaches to minority problems of blacks, Spanish Americans, Indians, and all the poor. Though the field of psychiatry has been strengthened and broadened by its association with social and behavioral sciences, mental health is now often confused with responsibilities for social conditions in which mental disorders breed ever more brilliantly. These include poverty, racial discrimination, unemployment, educational failure, and now we are asked to take into our special responsibilities the ethical problems relating to abortion, organ transplants and the like. Psychiatrists themselves are pulled in many directions, and some join in the clamor for instant results in condemnation of traditional methodology because results have been slow in coming.

The enormous demand for health services, including psychiatric, is discrediting all medical methods of treatment, and the necessity for trained personnel, and the adherence to high standards, while glorifying the untrained, and as many say, the acceptance of superficial efforts as the best that we can do at this time. Medical education is placing a demand for reorganization and shortening of the time required. This, and the assignment of more elective time serves to increase competition for the attention of medical students and the inclusion of psychiatric skills and understanding for all students. The elimination of requirement for internship is going against the strong desires of many psychiatric leaders, who wish to remain a part of, and close to general medicine.

We believe that psychiatry is strengthened if it is a part of the total medical picture, and will be weakened if it becomes confused with generalized social welfare, rather than with medicine. I believe there is a danger that the discipline of the rigorous medical training of the past will be lost for all physicians, and especially psychiatrists, and that the really difficult four years of medical school will become easy, and its standards of performance lowered. Thus physicians will lose part of their hard-earned skills, and with it the fundamental reason that individual physicians have the confidence of their patients. This confidence has, up to now, not been decried or denied in all the criticisms of the medical profession as a whole.

A general weakness in our field is the relatively small effort being devoted to primary prevention of mental disorders, nor do I see any organized approach to what is frequently called *positive mental health.* Primary prevention demands the finding of causes and eliminating or weakening such causes of specific psychiatric disorders, in other words, the elimination of a disease; and we must know the cause or causes. Attack on these causes is usually not a responsibility of mental health professionals; rather people in the field of public health and the lay public provide the resources to conduct any such attack that can be justified by scientific information.

Positive mental health, on the other hand, is the development of a strong and resistant type of person who will not succumb to any appreciable degree to social deprivation, tensions, anxieties, specific assaults on one's self-image, self-respect, and self-confidence.[43] We must recognize that overwhelming conditions will be quite destructive to the healthiest person, and everyone has a breaking point. Without proof, we at this time assume that emphasis on eliminating genetic defects, or compensating for them, emphasis on healthy growth and development, knowledge of and respect for the common obstacles and frustrations of life and a strong component for the philosophy of living, which permits and tolerates one's share of frustration and disappointment are well-enough authenticated to justify strong support. The war has taught us that the greatest asset to avoiding a *mental breakdown* is provision of strong support from those on whom one normally depends.

As the causes for mental disorders appear to be more and more overdetermined, a Freudian term meaning *with multiple causes,* etiologies are more difficult to identify. Nevertheless, the search in this direction has been one of our weak points, and must be strengthened. Primary prevention waits for this advance.

I believe the proponents for psychiatry and mental health have been delinquent in organizing their considerable information and experience to present to the public well-balanced views on fundamental principles relating to our field. We have been inclined to keep quiet and permit public comment on our branch of medicine and psychiatric component of social situations to be dominated by extremists and ill-informed persons, who may be partially right, but confuse the public, less than constructive in their outspoken, dramatic and emotional statements.

A leading pediatrician, in discussing the future of pediatrics, said recently, "I am convinced that there is no single, simplistic monolithic solution to the problem of the delivery of health care. It has been most interesting to me in past months to note how many different kinds of people have become experts on this subject almost overnight; economists, reporters, medical students and interns, and even some members of the United States Senate, few of whom have taken the trouble to gather the viewpoints of those on the firing line, that is, the physicians rendering primary care."[44]

I must add that in my own opinion, many of the outspoken *authorities* on medical coverage and medical needs, have approached their studies with certain predetermined attitudes. They've always been successful in discovering evidence which has supported their position. We physicians and psychiatrists must avoid the human tendency to approach our side of these discussions with equally discrediting biases; and we must examine every comment, be it high praise or destructive criticism, to find the grains of truth which are probably there, and work to overcome the weaknesses that are exposed, while at the same time, rally our informational resources to overcome the misconceptions that damage our efforts.

Our community centers, and all that goes with them, which are so basic to our move toward adequate mental health services, are receiving both strong condemnation and strong support. Obviously, some are doing well, and others poorly, otherwise how can such diverse opinions as "The concept is great, reality disaster," and "A clear case of over-sell," be explained? Both of these are alleged to come from officials in Washington who are at the same time promoting these centers and acts as a source of money and of the regulations governing them. Official Wash-

ington may have its share of the best brains and the poorest
brains and the most biased brains that all of us observe around
us. And from the field come these comments, "The best thing
that happened to this country,"[45] and "The most advanced system of health delivery in the country today."[46]

Major problems of our centers include financing, which is dependent on a proper balance of federal and state resources, location of authority and responsibility, and the passage of suitable
laws and regulations, such as state-county laws of Pennsylvania,
mentioned previously. An important factor also is the proper
utilization of private resources. Statements concerning extremely
high costs per patient served, must be traced for confirmation,
and careful analysis and the determination to operate on a financial basis within reasonable distance of other forms of medical
care.

In working out these problems, which should take a number
of years, there must be liberal prescriptions of time, patience, understanding, cooperation and mutual assistance, hard work,
and hard-headed analyses of local problems, including the maintenance of standards. Manpower, minority and consumers' interests are, of course, always with us, and represent areas in
which much has been done, and must continue. Some of the numerous predictions of drastic changes review much that has been
in the picture for some time. But some startling prophecies are
made, like determination of the special field of child psychiatry, to
be taken over by *family therapists*. Why not the expansion of the
child psychiatrists' function since those problems are fundamental
in the family equation? Another peculiar prophecy is the elimination of the best trained and experienced person, particularly if
he is a physician and a psychiatrist, his place to be taken by *90-
day wonders* from the ranks of less-educated, *indigenous* workers,
protected by consultants. These suggestions are hard to take seriously.[47]

The point of view in which many share lies in the demand
that more and more unsolved social problems be dumped in the
lap of mental health, as they used to be into the state hospitals.
True, we have demonstrated the leadership and success in
moving ahead of the pack, but we cannot permit absentee land-

lords of the centers to dump their problems on the heads of these centers, especially without consultation or added resources being given. There is also a serious tendency on the part of some psychiatrists who boast of being liberals and move out into social activism. They are confusing their citizen's responsibility where their skills are no better than many other types of individuals with their professional skills and experience where their real competence lies.[48]

As Churchill said, in contemplating a carload of whiskey, "So much to be done, and so little time to do it." But in this case there is time, and we must be willing to move slowly if great gains are to be made.

It is my opinion that the changes in the direction and quality of psychiatric care, and of the opportunities and functions of psychiatry, have advanced by reasonable and logical evolutionary processes rather than by revolutionary movements from pressures, obstacles, and compromises. I believe we will continue to go more or less in the same directions in which we are now moving, remembering that these directions have been changing slightly from year to year, and we have been responsive, I believe, and faithful to our duty in observing such social changes. I agree with Busse, who said in substance, if we as a group remain flexible, and examine carefully the demands for change, yielding to some but not necessarily all such demands, our progress will continue to move in whatever direction the real needs of society will lead us.[49]

We see ahead the prospect of greater federal intervention which, because the federal government holds the purse strings, we must regard as inevitable, but we can influence these changes so they can be potentially useful. Let us keep in mind that the private sector of society which includes the greatest share of specialists and generalists in ours and related fields, and creates the force known as public opinion, will have even greater responsibilities and opportunities than we now enjoy and than is offered by the governmental sector to keep health and mental health progress in line with the best of current scientific knowledge. To do this, we must insist on appropriate authority at different levels constant with our responsibilities. We must insist on adherence to high standards of therapeutic care, and a major input into planning and administration by highly-trained people. Our responsibilities are to all the people, and we must share our authority and responsibility.

Let me close by referring again to Brooks and his optimistic hopes for science: "I do not think that the scientific enterprise is going down the drain. It will change, as science has always changed. It will respond to new social priorities, but, like an organism responding to disease, it will develop antibodies which will fight and finally contain excessive control by external criteria and, in fact, will transform these external pressures into new opportunities and new fundamental fields of inquiry. But I could be wrong!"[50]

BIBLIOGRAPHY

1. Blain, D.: *Magic Years in American Psychiatry.* Philadelphia State Hospital, Lecture Series to Residents, 1967-70.
2. Holton, Gerald: *American Journal of Physics,* 29:803, 1961.
3. Maisel, Albert: Veterans Return I and II. *Reader's Digest,* pp. 45-50, April, 1946; pp. 22-24, May, 1946.
4. Deutsch, Albert: *Mentally Ill in America,* 2nd ed. New York, Columbia University Press, 1949, p. 449.
5. Deutsch: *op. cit.,* p. 293.
6. Ridenour, Nina: *Mental Health in the United States.* Cambridge, Harvard University Press, 1961, pp. 104-107.
7. Adkins, Robinson E.: *Medical Care of Veterans.* Washington, Government Printing Office, 1967, p. 115.
8. Ridenour: *op. cit.,* pp. 104-107.
9. Ridenour: *op. cit.*
10. Blain, D., and Heath, R. G.: Nature and Treatment of Traumatic War Neuroses in Merchant Seamen, *International Journal of Psychoanalysis,* 25:142-146, 1944.
11. Deutsch: *op. cit.,* p. 469.
12. Menninger, W. C.: *Psychiatry in a Troubled World.* New York, Macmillan, 1948.
13. As shown in the work of the Academy of Religion and Mental Health, New York.
14. Blain, D.: Survey of Extent and Distribution of Psychiatric Skill and Experience in the United States and Canada. *The American Journal of Psychiatry,* 109:10, 1953.
15. Goldston, Steven E.: *Concepts of Community Psychiatry: Framework*

of Training. Public Health Service Publication No. 1319, Washington, D.C., Government Printing Office, 1965.

16. Author's personal estimate.

17. Report of Mental Health Survey, State of Iowa. Washington, D.C., American Psychiatric Association, 1956.

18. Blain, D.: Peaks of Vision in American Psychiatry: a Personal Reminiscence. *Rhode Island Medical Journal,* 41(8):419-421, 1958.

19. Lewis, Benjamin J.: *V.A. Medical Program: Relationships with Medical Schools of United States.* Washington, Government Printing Office, 1970.

20. Blain, D.: "Novalescence," Presidential Address. *American Journal of Psychiatry,* 122:1, 1965.

21. Deutsch: *op. cit.,* p. 449.

22. Blain, D.: Private Practice of Psychiatry. *The Annals of the American Academy of Political and Social Science,* 286:136-149, 1953.

23. Gorman, Mike: *Every Other Bed.* Cleveland, World Publishing Company, 1956.

24. Stevenson, George S.: *Mental Health Planning for Social Action.* New York, McGraw-Hill, 1956, p. 9.

25. Boggs, Elizabeth: Development of NARC. Taped Interview with Daniel Blain, February 7, 1972.

26. Inter-American Council of Psychiatric Association: Report of Conference on "Mental Health of the Americas." Washington, D.C., American Psychiatric Association, 1968.

27. Appel, K. E.: Presidential Address. *American Journal of Psychiatry,* July, 1954.

28. Kennedy, John F.: Message from the President on Mental Illness and Retardation. H.R. Public Document, 88th Congress, 1st Section, February 5, 1963.

29. McNeel, Burdette: From Custodial Care to Modern Therapy Mental Hospital Institute. Toronto, Canada, January 21, 1958, Mimeograph.

30. Ridenour: *op. cit.,* pp. 104-107.

31. State of California: Mental Health Series Act. Short-Doyle 1957. And Lanterman-Petris-Short Act 1969. Department of Mental Hygiene, Sacramento, 1971.

32. Lewis: *op. cit.*

33. Glasser, Melvin A.: Mental Health, National Health Insurance, and the Economy. *Hospital and Community Psychiatry,* 23(1):3A, 1972.

34. Glasser: *op. cit.*

35. Blain, D., and Robinson, Robert L.: Personnel Shortages in Psychiatric Services, a Shift of Emphasis. *New York State Journal of Medicine,* 57(2):255, 1957.

36. Editorial: *Explorers Journal*, 42:129, 1964.
37. Brooks, Harvey: Can Science Survive in the Modern Age? *Science*, 174:21, 1971.
38. Haskins, C. P.: Science and Policy for a New Decade. *Foreign Affairs*, 49:237, 1971.
39. McElroy, W. D.: Editorial. *Science*, 175: 1972.
40. Stalones, Ruel A.: Community Health: Editorial. *Science*, 175:4024, 1972.
41. Kotin, Paul: Epidemics of the Future. Read at Philadelphia, College of Physicians, March 1, 1972.
42. Barton, Walter E.: Federal Support of Training of Psychiatrists. *Psychiatric Quarterly*, II(2):42, 1972.
43. Jahoda, Marie: *Current Concepts of Positive Mental Health*. New York, Basic Books, 1958, p. 7, 11.
44. Fischer, Carl: Pediatrics in the 70's. *Philadelphia Medicine*, 21:759, 1967.
45. Holden, Constance: Mental Health Centers: Growing Movement Seeks Identity. *Science*, 174(4014):1110, 1971.
46. Holden, Constance: Community Mental Health Centers: Storefront Therapy and More. *Science*, 174(4015):1219, 1971.
47. Rusk, Thomas N.: Future Changes in Mental Health. *Hospital and Community Psychiatry*, p. 1, January, 1972.
48. Kraft, Allan: Community Psychiatry. *Bulletin Menninger Foundation*, November, 1971.
49. Busse, Ewald: Future of Psychiatry: Hobson's Choice? Adolph Meyer Lecture, December 6, 1971. To be published in *American Journal of Psychiatry*.
50. Brooks: *op. cit.*

PART II
SOCIAL PSYCHIATRY

DIALOGUE WITH JOSHUA BIERER, M.D. THE ASSUMPTIONS, BELIEFS AND ACHIEVEMENTS OF SOCIAL PSYCHIATRY

PART I: Joshua Bierer, M.D. and John L. Carleton, M.D., Friday, March 19, 1971.

PART II: Joshua Bierer, M.D. and Norbert J. McNamara, M.D., Saturday, March 20, 1971.

I. DR. CARLETON: I would like to introduce to you my friend Joshua Bierer. Joshua is an unusual man. He has great courage and tenacity. He has great compassion and feeling for the sorrow, pain and frustration which are the by-products of human existence. He has created a theory and practice for social psychiatry, and he has devoted his life to his humanitarian profession. I had the very great pleasure of spending yesterday with Dr. Bierer. We traveled about town visiting some of the hospitals and psychiatric institutions; we spent some time in Robinson's and in the drug store across the street. I was simply amazed that with all these diversions, Joshua's most sincere interest was in the people in our community as he knew them and as he was getting to know them during his short stay here. He is able to focus in on individuals whom he has known for only a short period of time and to have a very sincere and vital interest in them as individuals. I think this is a very unusual and wonderful characteristic.

Let me also introduce our second panelist, Dr. Norbert J. McNamara. Dr. McNamara is currently the Director of the Santa Barbara County Mental Health Services. After receiving his M.D. from the University of Oregon Medical School and a doctorate in pharmacy from the University of California, he took his psychiatric training at Stanford University. He is especially involved in community psychiatry. He has previously been involved in day-centers, job corps centers, emergency room consultation services, and in the setting up of an honor farm as a therapeutic model. In Santa Barbara and in Lompoc he has established day-hospitals.

Together with Dr. Branch, he has developed a methadone program. Most importantly, Dr. McNamara has established mental health clinics in the downtown area and in the poorer sections of Santa Barbara so that the poverty and minority groups who suffer the most from emotional illness and social problems can get ready help in their own neighborhoods. Dr. McNamara will chair tomorrow's dialogue with Dr. Bierer and add some comments of his own at that time. We are most pleased to have him with us for the workshop.

Dr. Bierer was born on the 1st of July, 1901, in Radowitz, which at that time was a part of the Austrian-Hungarian Empire. Joshua, you lived there until you were fourteen years of age. When the First World War occurred your family fled to Vienna. There are a number of doctors in your family. Your father, Dr. Joseph Bierer, was an x-ray specialist; your grandfather, Dr. Reuben Bierer, was an eye specialist; your twin brother, Emanuel, a gynecologist; and your brother, Gideon, an orthopedic surgeon; your niece is an anesthesiologist; and her husband is an ear, nose, and throat specialist.

In the tribute paid to you at the time of your election as Corresponding Member of the Institute for Study and Treatment of Alcoholism during the Third International Congress of Social Psychiatry in Zagreb, Yugoslavia, this past September, it is recorded that during your early years of life you were frequently in danger. You said you trained yourself to accept danger as a part of normal living, rather than as something unusual; perhaps you can tell us why that was important.

Dr. Bierer: I was an awful coward as a child. You see, the first thing I ask from every psychiatrist is to be able to speak freely about his shortcomings and about the time when people considered him insane or mad or frantic or whatever you might call it, because I don't recognize madness. I maintain that the so-called sane society is not as sane as they think they are and the so-called insane people are not as insane as we think they are. We have obviously an interest in thinking that they are insane; otherwise we wouldn't be able to earn our bread and butter. Now, I believe that this is not an exaggeration. It is one of the fundamental beliefs of mine and a provocative statement which will probably be discussed by a number of you later. But please, before I start, I would beg you not to be sorry for me and to attack me with everything you have in you. You see, I am a masochist, and I enjoy that.

Just to finish your question. Being such a frightened child, I couldn't stay in the dark by myself. I was a very neurotic child. My father called all the doctors in town and I swallowed all the medicines available and obviously nothing helped. I suppose my whole theory of treatment is influenced by my own experience. At the age of fourteen and a half to fifteen, after we fled to Vienna when the Russians occupied our town, I was suddenly faced by my friend who said: "You come and join us; we are starting a new scout movement and you take over the youngsters of age eight to ten." Suddenly this stammering, frightened boy with all the neurotic symptoms was faced with a group of a hundred youngsters, all rowdies. What could I do? It was a question of just drowning, of running away, or of facing the situation. I learned how to stand up for myself.

Later on I went to Palestine. I lived in a kibbutz and worked hard to build a community. During this time I was often in danger, I was shot at. All these things made a man out of the neurotic, frightened child. I mention this because I think that facing a situation is an important factor in the treatment of difficult or maladjusted people.

DR. CARLETON: Josh, in 1920 you became acquainted with Professor Alfred Adler, one of the three pioneers of modern, dynamic psychiatry. You became his pupil, and you were analyzed by one of his students, Dr. Alexander Neuer. Can you tell us something about your experience with Dr. Adler?

DR. BIERER: Yes. Adler was a very great man which, I believe, future historians will find out. It was unfortunate that he grew up in the shadow of another great man, Sigmund Freud. Most people don't know that what brought about the rift between these two great men was an article which Adler published in 1908. It was the first time that one of the members of the psychoanalytic school published a paper on aggression.

Adler is generally known for having formulated the ideas concerning the *power complex* and *inferiority complex,* but this is a

misunderstanding. What Adler drew attention to were the social aspects of dynamic psychotherapy; and from that point of
view one can call him one of the fathers of social psychiatry.
Adler considered everyone a member of the whole community.
Unless the therapist can help the patient to feel that he is an
equal member in the community, he can never succeed in helping
him. *Adler said that the patient is a human being like the thera-*
pist. Adler was against the patient's being in any unequal position. The patient had to sit on the chair like the therapist.
Unlike in original individual psychoanalysis, the patient was
allowed to have social relationships with the therapist. Adler
treated the entire family. He urged us to see not only the family
but all people who are important in a patient's life, his boss or
foreman, the maid or anyone else. Personally, I like to see all
people, family or not, who are of importance to a particular
patient. These are some of the aspects Adler introduced.

Adler made another fundamental statement—that he did not
recognize mental illness. He gave me my first schizophrenic patient in 1925 and insisted that I must see in him just a human
being. I was to forget that he was schizophrenic. I must say this
helped me tremendously. Without Adler's guidance I would never
have done it and I would never have started thinking in the
right direction.

DR. CARLETON: Josh, what do you think about psychiatric diagnosis in general?

DR. BIERER: You see, I am a bit frightened because we have
some very important members of the APA here.

DR. CARLETON: A physician makes a diagnosis and on the basis
of a diagnosis proceeds with a form of treatment, or method of
treatment, which is fairly well delineated in advance. Why is
that method impractical in psychiatry?

DR. BIERER: Because, I am sorry to say, in my very considered
opinion, psychiatric diagnosis as it stands today is not worth the
paper it is written on. I'll try to prove it to you by telling you
about an experiment I published many years ago. In 1938 when
I started to work in my first mental hospital in Great Britain, I
came across a woman who, the superintendent insisted, was so
violent that he had to transfer her to the refractory ward. I

don't know what you call it here but the refractory ward holds people who are more violent and sicker than anyone else.

In studying this case, I found the following factors which are of importance. I found out that this girl came from the country to London. She was a very lively, very active, good looking girl. At the age of eighteen after she came to London she got a job in a block of flats, where she looked after members of Parliament and members of the House of Lords. They were all very nice, cultured people; they all liked her and she had a very good time; and not just with them, you know. She went out dancing every night and she enjoyed her life. But none of these many men whom she danced with proposed marriage to her, with the exception of one little man whom she called "the little worm." He was a plumber. He went on plumbing and plumbing his right to get engaged. She didn't take any notice. But the difference between him and the others was that he was stubborn—I believe that many women don't marry the men they love but the man who is insistent. So, in the end after five or six years she agreed to get engaged and after another two years she got married. And then, this girl suddenly found herself in a flat in the South End, in a little resort, away from London; in that flat she waited the whole day for the "little worm" to come home.

I think a big worm might be worth waiting for. But the little worm was a little bit too much for her. To cut a long story short, she tried to commit suicide. And she was saved and sent to a hospital. I did not know her then. But when she came out from the hospital after a time, she ran away from her flat to her parents in Wales. She was in her parents' home when her husband came after her. She tried to hang herself, but he succeeded in cutting her down and saved her life. Then she came to the mental hospital where I worked and my colleagues put a very lovely label on her as they put a lovely label on forty other women who were in this ward; the others were not all as violent as she. And the labels included everything with the exception of schizophrenia, that is, manic depressive, hysteria, anxiety, *et cetera*.

But I studied what was behind my patient's illness. I do not say that there are no physical causes, but where these have not been established I cannot do anything and it doesn't help me in my treatment. Therefore, I must handle those causes which I feel I can do something about: the person, the subconscious, the environment, the traumata, the whole upbringing, the childhood: the whole vertical and horizontal cut. Now you would expect if any diagnosis has any value, if it is somehow true, then you should have a specific treatment or near-specific treatment for each different illness, not in every case but in the majority of cases. But what would you say if you used one treatment for all the different cases with different diagnoses and this treatment achieved excellent results? Something must be wrong with the diagnosis.

Now this is what I did. I studied these women and found out that they suffered from about ten different things—they were all very active, you see, and that is why we didn't find any schizophrenics among them. They all had had a traumatic experience, generally with the father, in early childhood; they were all frigid. They got married because they believed they loved their men. In reality they used them as an escape from a situation with their parents which they could not bear. They were married and obviously didn't feel anything. They were unhappy, their whole life started to break up. Yet they did not have the courage to leave their husbands. Therefore, their only way out was to escape into a mental hospital. By understanding this dynamic process I came upon an effective treatment. The treatment was to take them away from their homes, to produce what I call a total separation treatment.

In the case of my patient, I talked to the husband and he nearly killed me. "You bloody foreign meddlers, I'll never allow you to take away my wife." So I had to disappear fast. But after she got worse, and worse, and worse, I went to see him again and said: "What do you think now about these bloody foreign meddlers, do you want her to stay in a mental hospital for the rest of her life or do you want to give her a chance? I must be very severe and impose this condition: that you have no contact with her whatsoever, neither by letter nor by telephone nor in any other way. If you don't agree I'll stop the treatment and you must get someone else."

If you believe in your method, I would say, you as a psychiatrist must be like a surgeon. A good surgeon, in a case of life or death, will not say: "Madam, I want to operate on you—now go home and think it over for a few months." A good surgeon will say, "Madam, I will operate on you this afternoon at two o'clock and if you don't agree, I advise you and your doctor to see another surgeon immediately." The same way, I think a psychiatrist has to make decisions if he is a responsible man and act according to his conscience. To cut a long story short, I took this girl to London. Mind you, it was more difficult to persuade the superintendent than it was to persuade the husband. He was just going to send her to the refractory ward when this "mad continental" came and said, "I want to take her out of the hospital."

I said I would take full responsibility. I was lucky to be able to get her back into the job she had had seven years earlier before she married. I said to her: "You are completely free. You are not married. Come and see me every week. You work, you love, you do what you like."

She soon found that she was no longer eighteen. Even at eighteen she didn't find anybody to marry except the "little worm." Now at twenty-five, her chances were less. Now without my influence she gradually came to see: "My goodness, I have a man who loves me. He is at home waiting for me." So she stopped coming to see me at the outpatient clinic.

By accident, I saw the little man at a different hospital. I went up to him and said, "What are you doing? How are you?" He said, "I've been ill, I've hurt my hand." You see, I was not supposed to know what had happened to his wife, she just stopped coming. I put two and two together. If she didn't come to see me, she went to my competitor; she went back to the little worm. I said to him, "How is your wife? When is she going to have her baby?" He blushed and said, "How do you know? She just missed her period last Saturday."

So you see, psychiatry is one of the most exact sciences, not as so many of our colleagues believe, just something up in the air, nothing to put your finger on. But I say it is an exact science like a jigsaw puzzle. If a problem admits of only one solution you are dealing with the most exact science you can imagine. But, I add, you must be a good jigsaw puzzler. This is where I agree with our chairman who says that psychiatry is a combination of science and art. Unfortunately, in our profession we have either scientists or artists and we need a combination of the two.

I almost forgot to tell you the most important part. I followed up this woman years later. She was happily settled in Wales near her mother with the little worm and two children.

DR. CARLETON: If anyone in the audience has a question they would like to ask Dr. Bierer I think this would be a very good time to do so.

QUESTION: You say that a psychiatric diagnosis is not worth the paper it is written on. What do you do in a court case when the court requests a psychiatric opinion?

DR. BIERER: I do admit that you need to satisfy yourself and the court with some sort of diagnosis. But you know in Great Britain all the judges have the worst possible opinion about psychiatrists. Judges are practical people with tremendous common sense. But many psychiatrists come in court and put a wonderful diagnosis—a marvelous label—to the court. The judge listens and feels inferior because he doesn't understand a word. And it helps neither the case nor the judge. (It might help the psychiatrist because he gets a fee.) I go to court very seldom but if I do I don't use a diagnosis.

Just to give you one example: I was asked to see a boy who had come before the courts and had been sentenced to ten months on account of some thieving. This was an appeal hearing. His solicitor asked me to see him. I did so and appeared at court. The judge asked me, "Doctor, do you come here to tell me that you can change this man?" I said, "No, sir." The judge, "Well, what do you want to say? Do you think that if he is given his freedom he'd be a better man and not repeat?" I said, "No. The only thing I can say, Your Honor, is that I have a big garden. My gardener is a former Army Sergeant Major. I think he can teach this boy some discipline that will make a different man out of him." I got the man off because I spoke common sense. If I had given a label to him I would have achieved nothing. I believe that the labels don't help us in court.

But you see, we psychiatrists in Great Britain have suffered from an inferiority complex for many, many years, and that is why we are trying so hard these last ten years to become consultants in teaching hospitals or consultants in other hospitals—to be on the same level with consultants in surgery or other medical specialities. We are trying to overcome our inferiority complex by trying to establish a system of diagnosis which appears to have a real foundation. If we are honest with ourselves, it hasn't a real foundation. A number of papers have been published (I can't give you the exact number) on patients who have been in various hospitals and received a different diagnosis at every new institution. The percentage of such patients is so high that you have the right to say that such diagnosis has no value. To come back to these forty women. I treated them with one form of treatment—total separation—and I had excellent results. With the exception of two women, they all went home and lived a happy, different life. They were able to feel, to be a good wife and a good mother.

QUESTION: Do you feel that there is any difference between a psychosis and a neurosis?

DR. CARLETON: Josh, I wonder whether it might not be well to define psychosis and neurosis if you would. These are terms which designate broad groups of psychiatric diagnoses. If you don't feel that psychiatric diagnosis in itself is very meaningful, what do you think about these two words?

DR. BIERER: I'll answer your question with a little joke. I love jokes, and I wish all young psychiatrists, social workers, psychologists, would take a special course in humor and jokes. And sometimes you can break the ice so beautifully—just with one little story.

Many of you know this story. What is the difference between not only a psychotic and a neurotic, but between a neurotic, a psychotic, and a psychiatrist? A neurotic is a person who builds castles in the air. A psychotic is a person who lives in this castle and a psychiatrist is the man who collects the rent. Now, *I don't believe in a difference between neurosis and psychosis,* although in practice we may differentiate between them. Some are frightened to commit themselves to a decision on these terms and in individual cases they say that this case is a borderline case. But where's the border? Which side of the border? What border? *etc.*

I ought to add that there are some cases that appear to fit completely into the picture of psychosis. But remember, for so many years we believed that you can't cure schizophrenia, it is incurable. If somebody cured schizophrenia or if the patient felt better we'd say, "Oh yes, that's only for a short time." And if somebody was well for a long time we would say that this was an exception. If somebody was well forever we would say, "Obviously, that wasn't schizophrenia."

Now, when you work in this field for as many years as I have and you try to be honest with yourself, you have to discard many theoretical positions you once held. I always tell my pupils and my assistants, "Forget everything you have read in psychiatric books, and especially forget what I teach you. Don't forget what you pick up when you watch me working with patients. These intuitions will help you in handling the patient more than all the theories could."

To return to the question of neurosis, psychosis and schizophrenia. I know I'm extreme, and people say that I am mad, and I know I'm a schizophrenic. But a schizophrenic as I see it lives in a happy world. I discussed it with a lady here yesterday. I said, "I awake in the morning at five o'clock and something comes into my mind—this morning it was a story—yesterday it was a new definition of psychoanalysis. I don't know where the idea comes from, you know, it's not connected with something from the day before or some discussion I had. It comes completely by itself and makes me feel up in the air. I feel wonderful, away from reality." And the lady, she is a sculptress, said to me, "No, you see for me, it's the opposite. When I create, I see reality better, in a different form."

Whichever way you interpret it, my feeling is that the schizophrenic lives in a world which is much nicer to him than our world and that is the difficulty of treating schizophrenia. It's a wonderful world because *he is creative in it;* of course, not in a practical sense. He creates his ideas, his illusions, his hallucinations, and he is very often very happy in this state. The difficulty is to get him out of this state and to get him down to this awful world. If one wants to, one can give a definition and say, people who are psychotics are completely removed from reality, they have no contact with reality. Neurotics are still living in reality, a distorted reality, but still reality. There is a difference of degree and not a fundamental difference. You might say that quantity changes over to quality at a certain point; then you might call the difference between neurosis and psychosis a qualitative one.

But these are all theories. When it comes to the practical application, to the treatment of schizophrenia, you have to study why this human being was forced to create his own world, why this world was too difficult to cope with. This is my definition of schizophrenia. You see, when I feel that life is too difficult for me I must escape, I might escape to mental hospitals. I might escape into illness or I might escape by creating my own delusionary world. If you look at it this way then you might have a chance to help the patient, because you then have to find out why this world was too much for this person.

Dr. CARLETON: Josh, you have given us a functional or operational definition of schizophrenia which holds that the person establishes an unreal world in which he can live when the environment is too difficult, or the family is too difficult, or the social world in which one was raised was too difficult. In Denmark, under the direction of Seymour Kety, some studies about identical twins are being conducted. The statistical records in Denmark are very good and the researchers are able to locate people even if they were illegitimately born and raised apart from their biological parents.

They are finding, interestingly enough, that there is more so-called schizophrenia, or more schizophrenic reactions, in those children who have relatives who have suffered from schizophrenic reactions or schizophrenia. The suggestion is that there is a genetic factor in schizophrenia. Do you have any feelings about that?

Dr. BIERER: Yes. In 1920, a German professor whose name I have forgotten found changes in the blood of schizophrenic patients. For a few years this change was accepted as a specific proof of schizophrenia. Unfortunately, a few years later some other researchers published a paper proving that these blood changes can be seen in so-called normal people, and this theory was given up. Now, I do not claim that there are no physiological, biochemical or electrical changes in the brain in any one of our patients. I can only say, until they are shown to influence the symptoms, I have no other choice but to concentrate on that part of the patient's life that I can do something about.

Point two, we don't know what schizophrenia is because there are so many different forms. I differentiate three forms and I'm sure that there are many others; but from the point of view of my treatment it doesn't make a difference if I make a distinction. For example, one of my first patients was an only child of two schizophrenic parents. The child was brought up in what I call *a social and emotional desert*. The parents couldn't show their love for her. They did not allow her to have any friends, no relatives, no one. Now this is a specific form of schizophrenia. And in these schizophrenic cases I have to reeducate the child step by step. Gradually, patiently I have to develop the patient's emotional and social life. In such a case drugs don't help me at all, except if the patient is very violent and I want to calm her down. And these cases are different, for example, from the schizophrenia which is caused by a number of unusual shocks, by traumata.

In my treatment I go by what has happened to the patient and try to overcome that particular point which was the cause of the patient's behavior. Mystifying words or phrases don't help me and I haven't seen any patients being cured by drugs. I've seen patients helped to live a more normal life by drugs, but I haven't seen that drugs really cured a patient. I have seen doctors who gave drugs and didn't know that they were good psychotherapists. We have one man in London who says he is against psychotherapy. But he's a very good psychotherapist without knowing it. He gets the confidence of the patient, he explores the family situation, but because he made a name as a leader of the drug theory, he's frightened to be caught at using psychotherapy. To come back to schizophrenia, I do not recognize schizophrenia as one illness. I do believe there are different escapes from the reality of life and you have to find out why that particular person had to escape and create his own world. Unless you are able to make this world palatable and give the patient the confidence to be able to cope with this world, that patient has no reason to come back to reality.

DR. CARLETON: I myself, Josh, have thought that all of us have the potential to become psychotic or that we are all crazy periodically throughout the day. This was one of Dr. John C. Whitehorn's concepts. He used the analogy of a sailboat which keels over in a strong wind. Some boats stay keeled over longer, others right themselves fairly readily. What we are talking about is an inter-relationship or an interaction between an individual and his environment. If this interaction goes wrong, we call the result *mental illness*. We might use the analogy of tuberculosis again. We call tuberculosis a disease, but pathologically what we see is the result of the interaction between the physical organism and the tubercle bacillus, for example, in the lung. The body throws out a protective scar tissue and attempts to isolate the irritant. The bacillus continues to grow and irritates the organism more which in turn throws out more scar tissue. What we're speaking of is really the result of an interaction between the body's attempt to fight against the trauma of the tubercle bacillus. What do you feel about these analogies?

DR. BIERER: I'm quite in agreement with that and would go a step further perhaps—and say that for me, medicine is a *Gestalt*. We must consider the body, the environment, the psychological relationships, that is the total picture. We must look at the total set up. This is what we call social psychiatry.

II. Saturday, March 20, 1971, began with Dr. Bierer being interviewed by Dr. McNamara. Dr. Bierer started by adding further information about social psychiatry.

DR. BIERER: At this point I should like to forestall some misconceptions about social psychiatry. Social psychiatry is not a school. I'm very much against schools although I know they are necessary for a certain time. They are no good if they force you to follow one particular party line, for science and slavery don't go together. You must be free to think, to exchange your views. Social psychiatry is a movement in which everybody has his own views. This, I believe, is very productive. I also don't think that psychiatry is a medical science. Perhaps psychiatry is a medical science, but social psychiatry is not only a medical science. We must have the courage and the honesty to admit that we psychiatrists alone cannot solve the problems of maladjustment. We must have a team, a team of equal workers. And members of this team are not only the people working in the field of mental health but the patients and the entire community as well. Now this is a problem on which there are different opinions in our field. Psychologists, psychiatrists and social workers will not be on speaking terms because we cannot agree on the question of competence. But we have no moral right to say that we want and have the right to teach people the science of human relationships if we can't agree among ourselves.

QUESTION: I am a sociologist with the Department of Mental Hygiene and I teach at the University of California at Riverside. From what you have been saying about mental illness I gather that mental illness might best be considered a myth—a useless myth—even a dangerous myth. Do you think that way of looking at mental illness is at all threatening to the psychiatric profession as we know it? and secondly, do you think that psychiatrists or mental health workers have a sufficient amount of self-confidence or mental health themselves to be able to accept this kind of threat?

DR. BIERER: Unfortunately not. And that is the reason why my colleagues think I'm an *enfant terrible* or that I am a man who lived much too long.

QUESTION: I'm sympathetic to Dr. Bierer's philosophy, but words like *total* always worry me a little. I can see how you have to state a new idea very forcefully and in such a way as to encompass all possibilities. But with regard to what really occurs are there not some patients who just have to be hospitalized? However few?

DR. BIERER: You are challenging an essential assumption. For forty years now I have been fighting to prove that mental hospitals are not fulfilling their job and are actually harmful. Why are they harmful? I have to bring that up before I come to your point. Why are they harmful? I believe they are completely against any therapeutic logic. Except for some cases, the majority of mental patients are people who cannot stand up to the pres-

sures of life. Therefore they escape from reality, from responsibilities, from a work situation and go back to mother's womb.

I believe with Rank that every person lives through what I
call a *North Pole* experience. I think we can imagine that when
we were a little baby in mother's womb we were in a most wonderful and warm atmosphere not interfered with by shocks.
Calm, quiet and I presume, not bored. But suddenly the baby
is thrown out into this cold world. I think we have the right to
presume that he experiences a shock which I call the *North
Pole* shock. Now it appears not illogical that when we meet difficulties in this cold world, we subconsciously want to rush back
to that mother's womb where we were protected and secure.
Therefore, I believe it is wrong to provide the patient with a
mother's womb which the mental hospital is. It is not always a
very nice womb, not the same womb that patients expected; it is
sometimes cruel, sometimes a snake pit, but still it is a place
where he can give up his responsibilities, where he doesn't need
to think, where he doesn't need to plan. But if you—any surgeon
would agree with me—if you don't move this arm for ten years,
this arm will die. Likewise every patient in a hospital who doesn't
need to think, to plan, to have any responsibilities, dies emotionally and intellectually. If you remove a person from the
community then he starts to die, because he doesn't have anything to do, to plan, there's no hope to live. That is why mental
hospitals are against any therapeutic logic. The exception, I am
quite prepared to admit, is the patient who needs a rest.

Now to your question. I admit there are a few patients who
are dangerous. But we made the majority of patients this way
by locking them up. The number of real dangerous patients
is minimal. With the right treatment very few patients are dangerous, but they might be dangerous momentarily. Of course,
with this belief comes one fear, namely that one day one of my
patients will walk out from my day hospital or your day hospital
and kill somebody. For then all of the community will shout,
"Lock them all up." I can understand their shouting but we
must make the community understand that they are unrealistic.

After all, I'm not asking the community to allow us to have a
higher percentage of murderers than the normal society. If the

normal society has one percent of murderers, why should all mental patients be angels. It's irrational. I can only say that in the over twenty years that I have been running my day hospital none of my patients has killed anybody or hurt anybody fatally. And I ask myself why not? We have the statistical right to have one or two murders (I don't know the exact percentage). The only explanation I have is that my patients were under supervision. Unfortunately we haven't got a system whereby we can examine the whole so-called normal population every morning and decide who is going to kill somebody that day and lock them up.

QUESTION: I believe it was Dr. Branch, yesterday, who talked about the distinction between being different and being dangerous. It seems to me that in our society, we as individuals are not sufficiently healthy to recognize this distinction and to tolerate differences. Therefore we feel impelled to put people away. Some societies are more tolerant. For instance, I read some anthropological studies on some African tribe. In one study a man was mentioned who thought he was a Greyhound bus. He used to run thirty miles everyday between villages, shifting gears, picking up passengers, and so forth. The children of the village would follow behind him and give him twigs and branches for fares. They would run for a mile and a mile-and-a-half and when they couldn't stand it, they fell behind and he would keep right on.

In their own terms, the people of the village considered him severely psychotic, yet they didn't feel impelled to put him away, to kill him, to isolate him or to treat him differently. They were willing to accept him as different. I wonder if this example doesn't say something about the community's need to have as much treatment or therapy as do patients. Perhaps until we come to the realization that nonpatients need therapy as much as patients, we will not have toleration for difference. It seems to me that this is one of the critical problems.

DR. BIERER: I agree with you that the whole of the community needs *understanding*—you don't need to call it treatment. We must ask ourselves why we meet such resistance from the community in understanding mental patients. I believe this is so because every one of us subconsciously has a fear of becoming mentally ill. This fear is as strong as the one we have of dying. Otherwise, I can't understand why throughout history we locked people who were different away, out of sight. And that subconscious fear of becoming mentally ill is very important for the intolerance we encounter from the community when we want to open a new half-way house, or a new hostel for mental patients.

DR. McNAMARA: Dr. Bierer, you probably saw from the last questions that, as we're beginning to implement social psychiatry in California, we have not nearly as many crazy people around as there used to be. People no longer have to act crazy when they can get treatment with a psychiatrist or at a hospital. Is this consistent with your experience in England?

DR. BIERER: Forty years ago when I said that madness doesn't exist, everybody wanted to lock me up. The superintendent of my hospital (who is a very good friend of mine) was very upset when I suggested that patients run the hospitals with us. That was in 1938. He was convinced that I was off my rocker. He couldn't understand my point then. Now he has accepted the whole theory because it worked. The great number of violent mental patients are figments of our minds—of our anxieties. We are creating them through mental hospitals. I am so happy that Dr. McNamara has found out exactly the same things we found in Great Britain. The majority of mental hospitals in Great Britain have reduced the number of their patients by half.

In two hospitals I know of, and there might be more, no patient has been admitted for the last three years. In the district where these two hospitals are located two psychiatrists cover the whole district—the mental hospital, the out-patients, the day patients—the whole thing. They're able to carry it out properly, and they haven't admitted one patient. My dream which I had for so many years is not a dream anymore; how far we can put it into practice depends on our courage and insight. Moreover, there are tremendous possibilities which we don't see yet—prophylactic possibilities. There are millions of women and some men who for one reason or another don't need to work and who are longing to give a meaning to their lives. They could help us with our work.

DR. HACK: My name is Dr. Hack and I am a private practitioner in psychiatry and I know we're here to talk about the movement which we all are a part of. Possibly this state is as much on the forefront as any other in the world because we have reduced our state hospitals. I think, though, we all too often refer to our ancestors as idiots and our heritage as worthless. I think that everybody needs to have a feeling that his heritage is worthwhile, that the people who went before him were not all idiots. The state hospital evolved, I think, out of a real need, namely that we didn't know what to do with the mentally ill. So, mental patients were retained at home until they became too great a nuisance and sometimes too great a hazard; and not necessarily from the standpoint of being a hazard to physical safety.

Modern psychiatry or at least effective psychiatry became available to a large number of people only as recently as the end of, or shortly before, World War II. With the advent of effective psychiatry we were able to begin to talk about no longer locking up people. And, there is a hazard of having ill people in the home. We used to say, and still say, when we see a schizophrenic young man, "If you think he's bad, wait until you see his mother." Schizophrenia as we were saying yesterday can be learned in the home. So our predecessors had a reason, I think, to "lock up" mental patients.

We no longer have the reason to do so and we're doing something about it. I see a schizophrenic young woman now whose mother had a very severe schizophrenic problem. The mother stayed at home because nobody in her community had any concept of how to treat her. She was retained at home until the community accepted her "being put away," which were the words used during those days. She was with her family long enough to quite mangle the development of my patient and of her brother who committed suicide. The brother could not survive this mangling and my patient is just barely managing to survive. What our ancestors did made sense in their own day.

To give another example: I have heard a lot about their sexual prudery—and yet I know that prudery itself grows out of a very terrible need; this has to do with the horrible problem of incurable and rampant venereal disease. It was so bad that they couldn't even talk about it. Sexuality was a dangerous thing along with the high mortality rates. Therefore to protect their families, the people developed these attitudes which we call prudery. I think now, with modern abilities to handle mental illness, we don't need to lock patients up.

If there's anybody that's not locking them up it's the State of California. The advent of the Lanterman-Petris-Short Act of 1969 was certainly not fought by psychiatrists, or not by very many of them. I think it's working—it's one of the biggest steps that any state ever made at any time for the advancement of the cause of the mentally ill. We moved patients to as near home as possible and we no longer banish them. Now I think as we begin to understand the socially ill, the prisoners in state prisons, we need to begin to work on their problem in somewhat the same way. I wonder if you'd like to reflect on that.

DR. BIERER: Dr. Hack brought out two very important points. One concerns community involvement in mental health, the other the treatment of social maladjustment. Let me speak about the first. You have some millions of people here whose life has no meaning and you have millions of patients who are considered ill and unable to work. The normal person—generally—only uses about ten percent of his abilities. A patient doesn't use ten percent of his abilities but sometimes nothing, sometimes one percent. Therefore, I believe that if we can help any patient to use ten percent or twenty percent or more of his abilities, this will help him more to take his place in the community than anything else. Drugs might be a help—but drugs generally are not a cure. A good part of helping a patient to self-determination and using his ability can be done by volunteers, but it must be done in the right way.

For example, years ago, I was invited by a few very nice ladies near Los Angeles to observe their work in a therapeutic self-governed club. I went and enjoyed the beautiful house. They said they had collected $35,000 every year for three years and had bought this house. In this big beautiful home there were about twenty wallflowers sitting along the wall—twenty schizophrenics. These lovely ladies gave them tea and cake and spoiled them. I was really in a very difficult position because these helpful ladies were the kindest people on earth. They thought they were giving me real pleasure by showing me that they had followed in my footsteps and had introduced the work which I proposed and carried out. I didn't know how to tell them that they did everything wrong. They copied the form but not the content of the idea.

The content of my idea is to use the principle of self-determination. The patient is not an object of treatment but a cooperator. That is the basis of the whole philosophy. If you use the principle of self-determination you not only save a tremendous amount of money but you give the patient enough confidence to take his place in society, to think, to plan, to work, to keep his family, to go out and meet girls, to get married or whatever it is. You can't do it with words alone. We brought about a revolution by saying that treatment on a verbal level is not enough, not that it is not necessary, but what we call experiential or situational treatment must be added to therapy.

A schizophrenic boy or a very lonely child might be in analysis for twenty-one years and he might understand exactly that he still lives in mother's womb, etc., but he will still not have the courage to get up and ask a girl to dance or to go out. You, as therapists, must produce situations in which, before he knows it he is on the dance floor and, too shy to sit down, he has to dance. In helping you do this you train your female patients, you don't need social workers. It's the first step, breaking the ice, which is so important. Now, may I point out your resources. You have a lot of gold, oil, minerals which you don't use—that is the patients themselves. Train your staff not to be too efficient. Train them to sit down and to read the newspaper or a nice book, to watch the patients, and to let the patients do everything. This is what I call guided democracy. I don't believe in the anarchistic principle of Maxwell Jones. I don't believe that it is useful treatment if you allow the patient to smash the place or to burn it. It might be helpful in one particular case, one particular time, to let aggression out, but to abreact all of the time is not good treatment.

You see, the great advancement of psychiatry or psychotherapy in the last twenty to thirty years is that we have developed a theory and practice which is specific to a patient's problems.

With some degree of certainty, if not with complete certainty, we can say that if we have a very shy person, the best treatment is group therapy and club therapy. If we have an obsessive, we probably can achieve results only with depth psychoanalysis—not in all cases but in many. In marital difficulties of a certain type total separation treatment is advisable. In the sudden form of depression, EST still might be very useful; not two hundred treatments as I have seen it, but three, four, five, or ten maximally. If we want to keep a patient quiet, certain drugs may be helpful. If we want certain schizophrenics accessible and if we can't do it otherwise, we can use tranquilizers.

We now have many methods which we can use to be more specific which we couldn't fifty years ago. But we haven't yet learned how to use the abilities of the patient successfully. I hope that you are going to do this during the next few years. Actually it's a trick you employ. The patient subconsciously wants to run away from all his responsibilities. We trick him into carrying responsibilities again. It's not easy. We need the guided democracy principle to get patients to do it. We just can't say "Go, do this!" Self-determination cannot be commanded. As a prophylactic measure we can use these millions of volunteers to do the work in the field.

Let me mention another concern of social psychiatry. We must work as a multidisciplinary team—that's the only way; psychologists, psychiatrists, social workers, patients, volunteers. We have created the International Association of Social Psychiatry for this purpose. We need local organizations which concern themselves with the mental health problems of the local population. In many local organizations professionals can help from behind the scenes. But we must be careful of fragmentation. That is our worst enemy. We must provide for one family a total approach —a comprehensive approach. That means that families not be divided up, today going to see one psychiatrist, tomorrow seeing another, the next day seeing a social worker. The total family must be under the care of one team.

QUESTION: I'm Mary Shaw and I work with the mental health program in the school district. I feel I'm caught right in the middle of a lot of confusion and I feel I'm caught with the kids who have the problems and a school system that does not really understand this problem.

In my job I am caught in the middle of conflicting needs and interests. Students are alienated from their schools and school administrators are angry at the students' boredom and hostility. When I attempt to make administrators understand the students' problems, they think I am crazy. School administrators try to find their own solutions to the students' problems without understanding the mental health implications. For instance, school administrators do a lot about curriculum and scheduling. We have a very sophisticated and flexible scheduling so that students don't have to sit in classes for six hours at a time. Students have a lot of freedom on our campus yet they are still bored and hostile to school. When you have an idea for doing something about the students' boredom and hostility, school administrators get worried because they are afraid you might foul up their curriculum and scheduling.

I hear that mental health people want to help kids with problems, yet you do not know anything about school problems. Yesterday Mr. Rozenfeld, the environmental planner, suggested that mental health people should not go to mental health meetings but to planning meetings. I am concerned that you don't go to school meetings. It is a tough problem for me. I understand the school practices and their mental health implications. But I do not get any help in dealing with the school people. My point is: shouldn't people in social psychiatry be involved in school problems and help us with school problems?

DR. BIERER: Yes, social psychiatry should. But you can't approach these problems by merely making some superficial changes. You must go down to the roots of the system and change the whole system. Several years ago I put forward a revolutionary idea. I was convinced that it would be taken up immediately because I thought it was a solution to a number of problems. I showed it to the British representative of UNESCO —he read it and said that it was an excellent idea. I said will you support it? He said, "Oh no, never!" I said, "Why?" He said, "Because, you see, you are providing a system which, when a dictator comes, is a ready-made tool to influence the entire community." I said, "Don't be a fool. If a dictator comes, he doesn't need a system, he can create it in five minutes." Let me tell you about this system. It applies in the main to Great Britain but you might have a similar situation over here. In Great Britain you have classes of thirty to forty pupils. I do not believe that any teacher can do justice to thirty or forty children and do justice to himself. Teachers are badly paid and you can't get the best people if you pay them poorly. Now, I propose that we should reduce the classes of thirty or forty to ten. You look at me and say that would be three or four times as expensive. And I say that it would be less expensive. Why? Because in charge of this group of ten will be an older brother. One of the pupils from fifteen to eighteen. What does it mean? It means that boys or girls from fifteen to eighteen who have no aim or motivation—who take to drugs—who don't know what their rebellion is all about, who don't know what life means—will have to be a responsible person to be in charge of a group, to form a family, a team.

Now it is likely that this treatment will give meaning to the lives of the boys and girls from ages fifteen to eighteen. In addition they will train in leadership. Ten of these groups will be in the charge of a trained teacher, who will be the mother or father. Assisting the mother or father you have a grandfather or grandmother, the best brains in the country who will teach large groups on television. Even the children in the most backward places will learn from the best brains in the country and also have the advantage of living in a family atmosphere. The children would be able to learn properly because this older brother would have time to give something to everyone. Different groups would be able to compete in games. And the teachers could be paid two, three times more than they earn today. I believe that this plan would solve many of the problems you brought up.

MARY SHAW: I agree with that but you see, you're now talking to people in mental health who understand your point of view. If you tried to sell your idea in the school, you couldn't do it because they would think you were not teaching kids.

DR. BIERER: But why couldn't you do it?

MARY SHAW: Because they wouldn't think that was teaching children.

COMMENT: How do you sell the school administration on your idea?

DR. BIERER: You see, my trouble is that I haven't even been able to sell it to you. As I watched your faces I realized that you thought I was crazy, as my superintendent did years ago. But I have to start somewhere before I can get the idea accepted internationally. Why is the idea not workable? Which people would not respond to it—the children or the population?

QUESTION: The school professionals are the ones with whom you have to deal. How would we implement it?

DR. BIERER: In a democracy we could create public opinion in favor of it by public discussions. That might take ten, twenty years, but we must get it started.

COMMENT: We could convince the kids and get enough kids who want to have such an education and they'll continue the revolution and force it.

COMMENT: But the schools don't listen to the kids—if they did we wouldn't have the problems we have now.

COMMENT: I think it could be implemented in the same way as the modular type teaching was implemented. That was introduced by getting the parents in the community and the teachers to back it. The teachers sold it to the school principals and to the community as a whole.

COMMENT: In the free school movement this has already happened. A lot of people have given up on the transformation of the public schools in their children's lifetime and they are creating free schools. In most instances these schools use a large number of people who are not *trained teachers*—they are using them in the capacity you describe. Through such a movement we will eventually transform the public schools when they lose too many students. And so I think what we described here is happening. And I for one have really given up (I have been a teacher for ten years) trying to do great things in the school structure. Public school administrators are concerned with maintaining the order of the system. I almost could not come to this conference. I teach history and sociology and therefore ought not to attend a mental health conference. If I had been a psychology teacher the school administration would have let me go without raising a question.

School administrators are concerned only with curriculum. They develop new curricula but they are very careful that by so doing they don't encourage students to do something weird, unplanned, spontaneous. Students on our campus last year painted a classroom. The teacher was given a bill for $700 because the administration had the maintenance people come and paint the room in the color usually used for classrooms. The students really painted the classroom colorfully—finest paint job ever given a classroom. So when students do change their environment—their way of doing it is not accepted. I've never attended a conference that has had the kind of impact, the kind of input that this conference has on me. I am being affirmed in what I do and at the same time I am being redirected to new tasks. It's a very beautiful thing—I'm glad I came.

COMMENT BY SPEECH THERAPIST: I am a speech and hearing therapist for the Santa Barbara City Schools. We have innovated in our schools a system similar to the one you talked about. Old, brighter or more understanding students act as student aides and help those fellow students who are backward in reading and other areas of learning. Student aides are not used on the scale you described but much change goes very slowly. I would like to suggest as Mary Shaw did that to bring about change you talk to more educators. Many of them would be willing to attend workshops such as yours.

QUESTION: I should like to ask a question to get back to an earlier subject, namely with respect to voluntary vs. involuntary treatment. On September 18, 1969, Thomas Szasz came down to San Diego and gave a talk on the myths of mental illness. He made the point that all the community mental health services— that is the hospitals—should be unlocked. One of the psychiatrists in the group became quite concerned about this, and he said, "Dr. Szasz, if we opened all the doors, we would lose half of our patients." And Thomas Szasz said, "Correct, for you'd have to be crazy to want to stay. But think of the good you can do with the half that remained." The problem I find is this: How

can we even help this half until we have completely open treatment facilities. In the treatment of the individual who goes into
the hospital we seem to be treating the person who comes in
labeled as *sick*. But we find that in the case of every hospitalized
patient there is a family member outside in the community who
is called *well*, and most anxious that the *sick* person in the hospital not get better. When the patient in the hospital gets well,
the individual outside does not stay *well*. How can we treat an
individual in the hospital separate from the family situation, if the
problem of *schizophrenia* is not a problem of individual X but a
problem of the individual within the family situation? How can
we help a person who volunteers for treatment when the rest of
the family refuses treatment?

DR. BIERER: But you always treat the entire family—including
the dog and everybody.

QUESTION: But how can you get unwilling family members to
volunteer—to participate even?

DR. BIERER: I have developed a very simple method which has
helped me to get any reluctant husband, father, son, daughter,
mother or relative who hates psychiatrists to come and see me. I
write a letter . . ."Dear Mr. Smith, as you probably know, your
wife has been under my care and treatment for such and such a
period of time. I am very worried about her, and I need your help.
I would be grateful if you would kindly come on Wednesday at
two o'clock. And should you not be able to come, would you be
kind enough to ring up my secretary to get an appointment."
Why can a man who hates psychiatrists not resist responding to
this letter? I just wonder what you think. If he loves his wife, he
cannot resist to come and help. If he hates his wife, he can even
less afford not to come. Why? He has many guilt feelings already
—how can he burden himself with more guilt by refusing to
help? It is really fascinating to see how such a simple measure
brings in these people. Once this man is in your office you, an experienced psychiatrist or psychologist, should be able to get him
to cooperate.

DR. McNAMARA: At this time, Dr. Bierer, I should like to summarize some of the elements of your philosophy and perhaps we
can conclude by your giving us your predictions for the future of

social psychiatry and the community. To many of us your philosophy may not now seem as revolutionary as when you started it in the early forties. Because of your own experience, your involvement with the scout group and the kibbutz movement in Israel, you focus your treatment on social and environmental factors in mental illness rather than on individual and interpersonal factors.

You tend to use a very practical approach. You deal with the patient's immediate problems and not with any theory or diagnostic classification. In your disregard for diagnosis you possibly upset some of your peers. In your practice of psychiatry you attempted to avoid the hospitalization, institutionalization of patients at all costs. You advocate the social rehabilitation of prison inmates within the community. You tried to keep people within the community, in their homes, on their jobs, with their families.

To achieve these goals you developed a number of different modes of treatment which include day hospitals, day and night hospitals with therapeutic community atmospheres. You developed self-governing social clubs, half-way houses; you used occupational therapy, group and family therapy. We are doing some of these things you do in England now in California. I understand that you in England now have more than two hundred day hospitals. I believe we in California have at least one in every major community. This has been due to your influence and that of Maxwell Jones who came here to San Mateo County as an early pioneer. He helped to develop this day center after which our Santa Barbara program was modeled.

To conclude this morning's discussion could you outline for us some of the present and future tasks social psychiatry will have to undertake?

DR. BIERER: Let me comment on a number of present day problems that I as a visitor to your country am concerned about. Your country determines so much of what we see other nations will do in the future, that you will, I hope, understand my remarks as a concern for all of us. Recently I was horrified to read a little book called *The American Health Empire* by Random House. I was horrified about many things but let me give you one or two examples. A ten-year-old boy was admitted to a hospital at 3:20 a.m.—he died at 11:34 p.m.—so he was in a hospital for these seven hours. His father received a bill for these seven hours. Can any of you tell me the maximum you can charge for seven hours?

ANSWER: $500.00.

DR. BIERER: You tried very hard but not hard enough. It was $1,717.80. . . . Another man was in the hospital for two months and received a bill of $22,147.95. He asked an independent doctor to look through the bills and this doctor wrote the following letter. I want to read it to you because I think there is a lovely, fine satire in it: "I do not challenge the indications for such an heroic form of therapy. But I am forced to conclude that few humans can survive such intensive care." Let me explain, in sixty days in the hospital the man had been given 1,100 laboratory tests. Now, after reading this book I got very worried that the wonderful Kennedy plan which provides a change from the locked-up mental hospital to community psychiatry will fail.

Since yesterday evening I have been a little happier because I have seen what Dr. McNamara and you here in California are doing. Maybe it is completely different from this book, completely different from what is being done in New York. Dr. McNamara told me that in New York they have four times as many patients in mental hospitals as you have in California—52,000—as compared to 12,000 patients here. I understand by next year you'll only have 2,000. That's wonderful. What has happened in New York is that they built new empires. The teaching hospitals acquired all the other hospitals, took hold of billions from the Kennedy plan and put it into so-called research and so-called teaching. The money which the legislators gave for the treatment of patients was used for research and training. Only ten percent was used for the treatment of patients. Now this is horrifying to me. I believe that this has to be changed.

The money that is spent for so-called research in this country is unbelievable. No where else in the world have I ever seen an institution like the Institute of Mental Health which has wasted billions on so-called research. Let me give you some proof. I went there and they asked me, "Dr. Bierer, would you like to have some money for research?" I said, "I'd be delighted." Well you can make an application. I then said, "I'd like to ask for $15,000 or $30,000." They said, "Don't be silly. We don't bother about such trifles. If you ask a half a million, we'll give it to you." I said, "But I don't want a half a million, especially not for proving that the form of treatment I have introduced, namely the community hospital, the day hospital, can save money. With the money you are spending here, you can provide excellent services for the whole of the population, not just for a few or for half of the population."

Let me also comment on the kind of research done there. They asked me, "Dr. Bierer, would you like to watch a treatment session?" I said, "I'd be delighted." Through one-way windows I watched a schizophrenic young man and his two parents. After two hours two psychiatrists came out and asked, "Dr. Bierer, have you any remarks?" And I said, "If you don't mind I have a question. It was very interesting, I watched it very carefully but it occurred to me that during the two hours not one of you two looked at the patient even once." "Oh," they said, "what have you seen?" I said, "Three times, I saw the patient making a remarkable movement when you or the parents said something." "Oh," they said, "that's very interesting, next time we must get somebody to watch from outside and write down the observations."

You see, they have conducted that research for five years and haven't thought of the simplest thing: that they have to watch the patient. You understand why I feel bitter? I'm not against research, you're doing some wonderful research—please don't misunderstand me, and it's a wonderful institution. But I bet any money that not five percent of the money they use for research gets results profitable for the patient—apart from drug research which is always excellent.

Now this is wrong. As long as you do not provide services for the total population, you have no right to waste so much. Let me make another point. You must settle the difficulties between you. You must get the members of the APA, I mean the two organizations both called the APA, to give up their defense mechanisms, not to be frightened—for a psychiatrist or psychologist who is frightened can't do his job properly—and work together as a team. You must be able to do that, otherwise you cannot educate the public, develop a real system of prophylaxis, change the false school system, change the prison system. If you cannot achieve unity among yourselves, I am afraid you are going to not only waste money but defeat the whole Kennedy plan of community psychiatry.

In isolated cases I can see reasons for optimism. Here in California you are trying for a community health program. Synanon is getting good results. The revolution of youth can be seen as positive. I am an optimist. I have seen some of my dreams come true during my lifetime. What does a man want more? But we still have to fight if we want to alleviate suffering. And with so much good will, you will surely find a way to improve your world and make it a society worth living in, unlike the society now where men are frightened, and wasteful, and intolerant.

Chapter 3

THE PRACTICALITY OF
SOCIAL PSYCHIATRY

C. H. HARDIN BRANCH, M.D.

SOCIAL PSYCHIATRY, like all scientific and clinical conceptions, must be viewed pragmatically as well as ideologically. And unless it improves the lot of those people we're calling the mentally ill, or the society in which *they* and *we* live, it suddenly will become a theoretical construct and an intellectual interest without lasting importance.

In essence, it involves the mobilization of all existing therapeutic forces for the improvement of those individuals who are incapacitated by their *difference* in a social matrix. Whether this incapacity is due to symptoms or to attitudes or to behavioral inadequacies is unimportant. A social psychiatrist deals with each situation as it is, not crippled by nosologic plaster casts which enforce certain procedures regardless of the terrain over which progress is planned.

The concept of social psychiatry is actually a return to an earlier *modus operandi* in which the *different* person, however he was designated, was regarded as a problem to be handled by his family and the community. Plato felt that the mad man should be kept at home with his family whenever possible.[1] Soranus, toward the end of the first century, described care of the mentally ill in terms almost like those Dr. Joshua Bierer uses. He felt that rooms should be free of disturbing stimuli. He felt that visits from relatives should be restricted, and I wondered if some patients might not feel that this alone would be a very good reason for staying in the hospital. There were discussions when the patient's condition permitted it. There were dramatic performances in which the patients participated, and there were group meetings.

The therapeutic effect of the community has been exploited by the town Gheel, Belgium, and its inhabitants since 600 A.D.,

77

when the shrine of St. Dymphna—the saint of the possessed—became a focus of interest for people who suffered from emotional difficulties. Even the existence of a modern hospital does not negate the influence of the town itself, and the vast majority of the patients are simply citizens of the community.

Institutionalization of the care of the mentally ill, in the broad sense of the word, began when the identification of mental illness with witchcraft and evil made the ecclesiastically organized society become a repressive force, although in its monasteries and hospitals some treatment opportunities did appear. Unfortunately, the taint of badness still clings to mental illness today and has to some extent clouded the treatment picture.

Progressive humanitarianism reappeared in the 15th and 16th centuries. An early writer, Cornelius Agrippa, was in the forefront of the attack on the cruel treatment of the mentally ill. Women's Lib might be interested in the fact that in 1509 he published a paper "On the Nobility and Preeminence of the Feminine Sex" and later risked his own life to save a lady accused of witchcraft. Better known in this area is Johann Weyer, who although he continued to believe in the devil as a vital force which did influence human behavior, adamantly opposed the concept of witchcraft and condemned the clergymen who supported a belief in it. He had really remarkable psychotherapeutic insights, and was most articulate in his exposition of the effect of kindness and understanding which the therapist must extend toward his patients. And he was extremely modern in the contention that the needs of the individual patients, rather than those of the institution, should be given primary consideration. No patient who has been awakened at 6:00 a.m. so the nurses could get their charting done before the shift changed at 7:00 could fail to be sympathetic with this idea.

In spite of these—and other—admonitions about the importance of the interreaction between the individual and helpful social forces, there was a general movement toward larger and larger institutions. Both here and abroad, the inexorable process was to the monolithic hospitals where quiet regimentation, polished halls, heavy rocking chairs and farms were the hallmarks. When one visited some of these hospitals it was interesting to note that the walls of the superintendent's office were often decorated with pictures of the cattle which had won prizes at the county fair.

The noxious effects of this institutionalization were dramatically demonstrated to me when I visited the University of Iowa a few years ago, and Dr. Paul Huston showed us two patients who were equally *ill* from a psychiatric point of view. One had been a patient *in* the hospital for so long that she had adopted a constant rocking motion derived from many years of sitting in one of the big rocking chairs lining the porches and halls. The other was a patient *of* the hospital, allowed home whenever her condition permitted it. While the reports of her home visits indicated a need for a good deal of tolerance from her family and neighbors, at least she herself was still alive, not a conditioned unit in a system. Ken Kesey has given us a poignant and tragic story of a brave man who almost succeeded in breaking the system by his own initiative, but most patients lack his fortitude and persistence.[2]

This institutionalization, part of what Reich designates as *Consciousness ii,* is almost inevitable with any gargantuan scheme of things.[3] Fortunately, at the moment there is a counter-current against it. By moving patients from their institutions to the communities we can take full advantage of the treatment and rehabilitation which are available from the healthy forces outside the hospital walls.

It's not going to be possible, however, merely to close the hospitals and move patients to the communities. The Lanterman-Petris-Short program in California is designed to facilitate this and in many ways this is being accomplished. However, the closing of some state hospitals proceeds side-by-side with the development of more halfway houses, adequate nursing homes, and other types of shelter. As we will see later, there still are patients who will need havens, but these can at least be part of their community picture and not of isolated asylums.

There are some additional problems we should examine. For one, it is essential to identify those which are directly accessible to mental health treatment procedures. Some problems simply are not. The person who says, "The world's a mess and I see no reason for being concerned with what others do with it" is simply dealing with reality in his own way. A recent survey of the people in Isla Vista, well-known suburb of Santa Barbara, California, showed that 76 percent simply felt a sense of alienation from the culture and no particular need to do anything about it. And as the well-known *New Yorker* cartoon has the psychiatrist say, "I would like to help you, Mrs. Glutz, but, as you say, it all seems so hopeless."

Some mental health workers are, I feel, overgenerous in their acceptance of problems. They have what I like to call the *Statue of Liberty Syndrome*. Like the lady in the harbor they say, "Bring me your tired, your poor, your huddled masses yearning to breathe free." But fatigue, poverty and political injustice are not mental health problems in the sense that they are accessible to specific mental health treatment approaches. And we can uselessly exhaust our energies if we do not differentiate to ourselves and our patients those things we can treat and those things we cannot. What's the *normal* reaction to the Vietnam War, the sociogonadal gap—which means that we can make babies earlier than we can make a living—the discrepancy between the propaganda about the SST and the lack of money for schools and slum clearance? If a patient says the whole business is psychotic, crazy people are in government and he's worried about it, what treatment can I offer him?

We are dangerously close to suggesting that any discomfort should be avoided and perhaps can be eliminated if we can obtain the proper pill. The pharmaceutical houses play into this when they suggest that dislike of doing dishes or mopping is a sign of emotional difficulty accessible to chemical treatment. In one advertisement we see a distraught, angered man who is exclaiming, "Women are impossible." At first glance we might assume that he is the candidate for a tranquilizer, but the message to the psychiatrist is, "In pre-menstrual tension your prescription of Equanil can help ease his wife's anxiety thus reducing her irritability and nervousness."

The procedure of treating one person by tranquilizing another, and the ethics of this suggest that many people feel that the pursuit of happiness is an inalienable human right and the capture of happiness highly probable. If we accept this goal for our therapeutic efforts we and our patients are doomed to disappointment because the best we can honestly offer them is the ability to choose wisely between relative discomforts. The sooner we make that plain, the better for everybody.

We can, however, approach our appropriate goals with considerable optimism. We do have, as the protagonists for social psychiatry point out, a smorgasbord of therapeutic possibilities needing only our imagination and energy to mobilize them for the realistic improvement of our patients. Many doors have been opened to patients and their families and we can utilize them.

Parenthetically we should note that we mental health workers do have a problem in society's demand that antisocial forces and people be restrained. There are those who feel that mental health philosophy permits, condones, or even encourages the release to freedom of individuals who have been aggressive and may again be *dangerous*. It is interesting to note that various rightist groups, including the John Birch Society, have accused the *Mental Health Movement* of conspiring to imprison people who are enemies of the movement. Either way, we're wrong! At any rate, it is certainly true that some individuals, for their good and/or the good of society, must be kept out of circulation for a time. History does, indeed, repeat itself; following the McNaughton decision in 1834, the London streets were filled with doggerel like:

> Ye people of England, rejoice and be glad,
> For ye're now at the will
> Of the merciless mad.
> Do they wish to spill blood
> They have only to play
> A few pranks, get asylumed
> A month and a day;
> And hey to escape from the mad-doctor's keys
> And pistol and stab whomsoever they please.

Short of these problems there are the individuals whose *sickness* is produced by diagnoses and the expectations attached to them. Emphasized by social ostracism, crystallized by intitutionalized management, and maintained by roles assigned and administered by those who gain from keeping things as they are, these diagnoses set in motion ever increasing incapacitation. And for these, the majority of the mentally ill, social psychiatry and smorgasboard approach provide a way out and back to full social participation. What is needed is love, imagination, and insistence on seeing potentials rather than symptoms.

In all this, the role of the therapist—whatever his or her professional background, training, or label—is preeminent, for the exchange between the therapist and patient provides the springboard for other social interchanges. Dubois insisted on the therapist's conviction that cure was inevitable. He said, "We practitioners ought to show our patients such a lovely and all-enveloping sympathy that it would really be very ungracious of them not to get well."[4] Dr. Kenneth Appel had this same quality; one patient at the Institute of the Pennsylvania Hospital told me it was easier to get well than to have Dr. Appel on your back insisting that you get well.

The therapist's activity is far from the *gray screen* concept traditionally assigned to the psychiatrist. Robert Knight said, "The patient can best make contact with somebody he is able to feel is like, or has been like, or could be like himself! I believe a therapist cannot convey this feeling to the patient unless he feels it himself. Optimism and liking for the patient go hand in hand as do pessimism and dislike for the patient and he responds accordingly."[5] This is recognized in another cartoon from the *New Yorker* in which the psychiatrist says to the patient, "I suggest you see another psychiatrist, Mr. Thatcher. After listening to your history I find I've taken an intense dislike to you." Perhaps the ultimate illustration is the often quoted story that Rioch had found a patient especially bright, alert, and interesting on five specific days; these turned out to be the days on which Rioch had himself taken amphetamine.

A special kind of therapeutic exchange occurs in many communities in which certain key individuals rapidly assume the roles of confidants or advisers and markedly contribute to the mental health of their neighborhoods. We found this true in a door-to-door survey of mental illness in Salt Lake City. We even wondered if it might not be possible to identify these people, offer them some training, and find out if the incidence of mental illness in a neighborhood or a community could be favorably altered by their efforts. One could, of course, guess that training might diminish, rather than improve their effectiveness, but this could also be assayed.

However we do it, we must see to it that the interreaction between the person and his environment is a helpful, not a hurtful one. We must see to it that the *different* person is not always thought to be a *dangerous* person. After all, we psychiatrists have been called *alienists* for years. Margaret Tsuda said:

> There is a theory
> that holds every
> verbal exchange from
> casual/impersonal
> "Pardon, is this a bus stop?"
> "Yes, it is."
> to ardent/ personal
> "Dear heart, will you marry me?"
> "Yes I will"
> to be a sort of transaction—
> a mutual exchange
> between parties of
> first and second part,
> If so
> it behooves us to be
> good businessmen all day
> giving fair weight to
> every question asked
> making sure that
> our answer fits
> our customer well.
> And never pocketing a
> cheery greeting
> without
> payment in kind.[6]

Earlier I said we should give some thought to diagnosis. There are those who feel that diagnosing is stultifying and even dangerous, in that it pigeonholes people and to some extent de-

termines not only how we regard them but actually how we
treat them. Nowhere is this more true than in the group of conditions we call the schizophrenias. There is far too great a tendency to think, once the label has been attached to the person,
that we are dealing with a hopeless and deteriorating situation,
that the person *has* schizophrenia, with the implication that he
will not be able to rid himself of his schizophrenia. I find it useful to remind myself that we should use a verb rather than a
noun concept in dealing with the problem—actually, something
of this sort is implied in our talking of reactions rather than
conditions.

By this, I mean that what we call a schizophrenic is a person
who is *schizophrening*, but some have to continue *schizophrening* indefinitely. It is true that some start *schizophrening* earlier,
start doing it with less stress than others, have more difficulty
stopping it and so on, but there is almost no person who cannot,
if the need arises, stop *schizophrening* long enough to cope with
an emergency. It is our task to mobilize social and personal forces
to encourage problem-solving by methods other than *schizophrening*.

An important part of this mobilization of social forces is our
attitude toward work and leisure. Our elders have been responsible for providing us with such aphorisms as "Satan finds some
mischief still for idle hands to do," and "Anything worth doing
at all is worth doing well," and "The idle hand is the devil's workshop." It is true that productive, rewarding activity is healthy
and health-giving, but activity qua activity is not. The man who
is job-oriented, like the woman who is uterus-oriented may have
a great vacuum when these orientations are no longer applicable. Retirement can lead to the corrosive effect of boredom if
we are not prepared for it.

This is an area in which social forces can be prophylactic, as
we prepare ourselves for the shorter work week, the earlier retirement, and even the contemplative kind of activity which is
somehow suspect in our busy world. Anyone who doubts that
quiet is suspect need only sit quietly in his living room not reading, not watching television; within minutes family members will
conclude that he is either ill or angry. We need some reassur-

ance that *being* has value. Sartre, among others, has reminded us that the process of being involved in something is more important than the nature of something.

The philosophy of social psychiatry, then, means taking a long and careful look at existing methods and institutions for dealing with the problems of those people who are called mentally ill, and remaking them and enriching them by the use of social and personal forces outside these institutions. Merely relabeling is not sufficient, but a truly dynamic search for the healthy forces available in patients and the therapeutic environments can change the total situation.

There probably should be a word of caution about the use of nonprofessionals. Many people have instinctive abilities which, as noted above, might be hampered by structure. But this is like trying to develop a beautiful garden without using an expert. We can love flowers and hate weeds and some of us have naturally green thumbs, but it may also be useful to call in a professional gardener once in a while.

What pervades the whole field is the excitement of a new course, historically respectable but with new applications. The victims of the accustomed ways will have cause to be grateful for these efforts. The only danger is that social psychiatry may itself come to be institutionalized, and this would be sad. The revolutionists' barricades of yesterday can be the roadblocks of tomorrow. It is true that meetings require organization, as does the network of therapeutic activities, day/night hospitals, outpatient clinics, lodge-type living situations, recreational possibilities and so on which this new philosophy envisions. All this can be facilitated by organization if the organization can be prevented from freezing solid. Whatever happens, the concepts in social psychiatry must continue to be the juices in a living, breathing entity. They must never be allowed to turn into embalming fluid.

BIBLIOGRAPHY

1. Plato: Dialogues of Plato, *Laws*. Book 11, Great Books Edition, Chicago, University of Chicago, 1952, vol. 7, p. 782.
2. Kesey, Ken: *One Flew Over the Cuckoo's Nest*. New York, Signet Book, The New American Library, 1965.

3. Reich, Charles A.: *The Greening of America*. New York, Random House, 1970.
4. Dubois, Paul: *The Psychic Treatment of Nervous Disorders*. Trans. Jelliffe, Smith Ely, and White, William A., 4th ed. New York and London, Funk and Wagnalls Company, 1908, p. 226.
5. Knight, Robert P.: Presidential Address. *Psychiatry*, 9:323, 1946.
6. Tsuda, Margaret: Transactional Analysis. *Christian Science Monitor*, p. 8, Feb. 23, 1971.

PART III
PLANNING FOR THE MENTAL
HEALTH OF THE COMMUNITY

Chapter 4

ENVIRONMENTAL DYNAMICS: MARY HAD A LITTLE LAMB WHO DIED OF EMPHYSEMA

LOUIS L. ROZENFELD

PROMISE A LOT; deliver a little. Convince the people they will be better off, but do not implement dramatic plans. Try new programs, each interesting but marginal in impact. Avoid at all cost —in more senses than one—any attempt to carry out solutions comparable in size to the problems at hand.

Have middle income civil servants; hire upper class radical students to use low income minorities as leverage against the political establishment. Complain about students going around disrupting things and chastise big business for not cooperating with those out to do them in.

Feel guilty about the poor people; act surprised they have not revolted before; express horror when they follow your advice. Push a little, feel guilty again; alternate with a little suppression, mix well, apply a match and run to your local psychiatrist.

Our neurosis is exquisite; we all play the game and leave the couch worse off than when we started. We get hooked on symbolic issues. When we fail, we get the shaft and are revealed as useless. If we win, we still get the shaft because it is soon clear that nothing has changed!

We, urban animals, have been crooning the *environmental blues* lately; we feel bad and frustrated. We know the environment is crumbling, that the sky is about to fall in, but we can't think of anything to do.

It is like the fat woman asking her doctor how to quickly lose twenty pounds. "Cut your head off," he says . . . we want to, but where is the head? Where are we? And how in the hell did we get there? Well, let's put a bit of historical perspective on the problem.

The Past

Some philosophers contend that Adam and Eve were expelled from the garden of Eden, not for eating the fruit from the tree of knowledge, but for casually throwing the apple core on the ground, thus inventing pollution. Adam was reported to say, "Eve sweetheart, we are now living in a period of transition. . . ."

This incident happened some time ago. Actually, scientists tell us that our world is five billion years old, that we have been on earth for some 250,000 years and that we, homo sapiens, started to record history some five thousand years ago. Yet, all but a few of the products and materials shaping our environment today, have been created in the last hundred years! The most significant technological advances of our day, automation, computers, nuclear energy, television, and many more have been developed in the last forty years! The telephone, the skyscraper, the incandescent lamp, the automobile, the elevator, did not exist a century ago! If we equate the earth's history to a book of a hundred million pages, five miles thick, our contemporary technology would be but the last page! If we equate man's five thousand years of recorded history to a hundred lives, our modern world would be but one life span!

We have not taken enough time to analyze what the misuse of our new marvelous technology has done to our environment, to our community, to our health. Fifty years ago, the importance of the environment was something people read about in the works of Emerson and Thoreau. It was a delightful and inspirational experience, intellectually rewarding, but of no apparent practical application. Urban children learned about the wonders of nature secondhand, and our urban parents dreamed of cool green forests and rippling brooks to replace their hot and sticky city's environment. In the country, rural parents cursed the forces of nature for making their lives difficult and had little taste for natural beauty. A tree was something to be cut down to make lumber for a house! At the same time, our industrial, economic, and urban population explosions attacked the environment with vigor, gobbling-up nature as a matter of course. The name of the game was progress and efficiency and prosperity. Seemingly, no one cared.

We dumped smoke into the air because there seemed to be plenty of space to absorb it, and as a matter of pride, communities pointed to chimneys belching smoke into the atmosphere as evidence of industrial activities and prosperity. We poured our industrial waste and our city sewage into streams because it was the easiest, quickest and cheapest way to get rid of it, and little thought was given to the consequences. We built highways, transmission lines, pipelines, and other evidences of industrial advancement with carefree abandon, and with little consideration for any other than the Euclidean principle that a straight line was the shortest distance between two points. Still no one cared, until fairly recently.

Now, we are experiencing a period of unprecedented affluence, but now we know affluence is not enough. We have reached great technological achievements, but now we know technology is not enough. We must think more about our future—our future as human beings. It is truly a question of survival, our survival. Well, let's pause and ask ourselves what is going to happen on the next page, in the next life span, the short thirty years remaining in the twentieth century.

The Future

Twenty years ago, nuclear energy was used only for destructive purposes. Today, we are using this energy for power generation, for curing dreaded diseases, for converting sea water to fresh water. Soon we will be using it to move mountains and to dig canals, to bring life and civilization to arid areas.

Our oceans cover seventy-five percent of the earth's surface; they possess virtually inexhaustible food resources and more mineral wealth than we could dream of. Yet, we know less about the bottom of the sea than we know about the surface of the moon.

During our children's lifetime, medicine will have a cure for most of the known diseases. Life expectancy will extend, maybe to 120 years! Proportionately, our productive working life will also expand. Our creative geniuses, our Einsteins of the future might be able to work productively for one hundred years!

Psychokinetics, or the control of mind over matter, will some day be a reality. Crazy? Impossible? Well, the airplane and dozens of other ideas at their conception were *proven impossible and absurd* by renowned scientists.

The Present

But let's get down to business! Let's relate progress to the present problems, to our city, to our people. People are dynamic; they change, and today, the most talked about change affecting our environment is our population explosion. Yes, by the time we finish our meeting today, there will be 100,000 new human beings born in the world. Yes, the world's population will double by the year 2000 from three billion to six billion!

By the year 2000, we will be consuming as much power in one year as mankind consumed since we harnessed electricity! By the turn of the century, we will build an inventory of homes, hospitals, parks, and factories equal to the entire inventory accumulated on this continent since the pilgrims arrived.

Yet, the problem is not more people; we have plenty of room and plenty of resources, the problem is too high a concentration level of population. In the United States alone each year, one million acres of our countryside are converted to urban development. In twenty years, we fully expect that ninety percent of the United States population will be living in gigantic metropolitan areas, and we already know what this can do to our community health and to our environment.

Our environment—which in our urbanizing world really means our urban areas, our cities—is more than a technical definition, it is the expression of our values . . . it is a complex living entity to which each and every human being contributes.

The architect with his discipline contributes to it, as does the physician. There is also the landscape architect, the statistical analyst, the economist, the sociologist, and the political scientist, to name just a few of the professionals who bring their knowledge to bear on the complex problem of our environment. Each of these professions is committed in its own way to the solution of our problems . . . but the requirements of our communities are such that no single discipline, no single profession, no matter how sophisticated in its own right, is equipped to deal with all of them, and when you attempt to make them work together, you have got yourself a problem.

I read a few pages of an old history book the other day, and it told about Moses trying to get out of Egypt. With the Egyptians in hot pursuit, Moses and his people approached the Red Sea. Desperate, they turned to their leader for guidance and Moses told them of his plan—somehow the waters had to be parted. But immediately, Moses was told "it cannot be done."

The city planner said: we've got all kinds of problems, Moses. First, water must go somewhere; it will flood the country roads, over-tax the drainage system, flood the farmlands and destroy the crops. Second, the bottom of the Red Sea will be muddy and full of pot holes. It will be impossible to travel, and worse it will be economically unfeasible. Further, the existing zoning ordinance does not permit the use of the Red Sea.

Then came the ecologist; he had no interest in the economic feasibility, but he did not think that it would be ecologically desirable. He said it will disturb the ecological balance, that microorganisms will die and interrupt the chain of life. The environment will be irreparably damaged. Thus, he must recommend against it.

The attorney said: I have made an exhaustive search of the law on this subject, and based on the previous reports, the damages would be tremendous. My research shows that in Cairo 24:16 Noah versus the Lord that you, Moses, must bear the responsibility for these damages. It also reveals that your potential liabilities far exceed the limit of your insurance coverage. I must recommend against it . . . in addition, Moses, I don't think I can get you the thirteen votes of the Red Sea Conservation League.

The psychiatrist then took the stand: impossible Moses; the shock of seeing water parted will create such neurosis in the ranks of our people that they will not be able to function as normal human beings for two or three generations. Further, we don't have enough psychiatrists to take care of all the cases that would come out of such an incident.

Unfortunately, the last page of the story was missing, so I still don't know just who suggested it, or how Moses arranged the divine intervention that parted the waters.

Now, in a way, we today are in the same situation, in that we have many people advising us as to what we can or cannot do. We have demands and schedules breathing down our necks, and sometimes our problems seem to be just as big as those that faced Moses. There are many times when I know I have hoped that I could have some divine intervention. But, until that time comes, we must very intelligently tackle our problems ourselves.

Well, enough preaching; enough telling you how we are poisoning our skies and how bad the water tastes in my house. Let me give you my ideas as to what we professionals can do about our environmental problems.

Some Recommendations

FIRST, WE PROFESSIONALS MUST COOPERATE. In our environment all organisms and all systems are interdependent. In our complex and beautiful world, it is no longer possible to attack a problem or identify the success of any endeavor with any one profession. Specialists should seek support, advice, and help from other professionals, early and continually in all their endeavors.

We have more than a professional responsibility to our environment. *We have a commitment:* a commitment to build and develop our environment in such a way as to achieve excellence, and to satisfy human needs to the fullest. Only the human mind will solve the world's pollution and environmental problem, and not the genius of one particular profession alone. Engineers, architects, city planners, physicians should meet and confer with other professions to learn and comprehend other viewpoints, other value scales and judgment techniques—just as we are doing today. We must learn to ask other professionals not to work for us, but with us. We should not become *instant experts* at other professions, but sincerely appreciate and seek the support and cooperation of other disciplines, foreign to us as they may be.

Once a very sad animal, a useful animal, who destroyed vermin and improved the ecological balance of nature, went to a wise old owl for advice. "Why am I so hated and shunned? I love people; I want to help them, but they don't like me! What can I do?" The wise old owl thought for awhile and said, "change yourself into a beautiful flamingo. Then you can stand in a beautiful reflecting pool, on one leg, in the middle of the painted desert, and everyone in the world will come to see you, admire and love you." And that poor, sad animal said, "But wise old owl, how do I do that?" and the wise old owl answered, "Don't ask me, I am a psychiatrist—that's a detail to work out with an environmental designer!"

SECOND, AND ABOVE ALL, WE MUST KEEP OUR INTEGRITY. The market place seeks advice and guidance and direction from its consultants. We should give our client what he needs, and not simply what we think the client wants. This should be the basic credo of all professional integrity. The client, the community, the various professional objectives are not to be viewed as *conflicts* but as *different points of view* toward the same problem or opportunity.

The role of any professional is not to ignore, but to coordinate these various initiatives and personalities; not to restrict, but to encourage expression and differences of opinion. The objective of any professional is not to design his own particular hardware system, but to make sure that whatever system it might be, it will upgrade the level of life quantitatively and qualitatively alike.

THIRD, THE WHOLE IS MORE THAN THE SUM OF THE PARTS. Professionals dealing with hardware, such as engineers or constructors, must become sensitive about environmental problems in a much broader sense. They must develop a humble understanding of the social, ecological, and mental forces affecting their clients, *our clients, our communities.* In parallel, the soft professions, medicine, sociology, anthropology, must also develop a deeper understanding of the economic and quantitative requirements of the market place.

A phenomenon seldom recognized is the vast interrelationship of elements of community health. What an architect designs or a physician professes in one corner of the environment will have ramifying effects throughout the entire physical, social, political, and economic fabric of our community. It is no longer valid to take the position that results are achieved as long as they are economically feasible, and to ignore nonrevenue items such as aesthetics or well being. What happens in Santa Barbara affects Watts; what happens in Watts affects Washington, D.C. The whole urban world is one complete total system.

FOURTH, WE MUST LEARN TO COMMUNICATE. Having been involved in the field of environmental planning for the past few years, I have had an intensive post-graduate course on the subject of communication with experts, instant experts, and real experts. In general, as any large multi-million dollar endeavor approaches completion, it is going quite smoothly. As the public can see with their own eyes what this particular project will do for them, they are far more able to judge for themselves its value or failure.

However, in the initial phase its value is not evident: there is a great *sound and fury* and many suggestions are made for far-out schemes. Inevitably, one or two people are quite violent in their public statements, that they alone know what is best, that everything is being done wrong.

Earlier in my career, my response to false or inaccurate comments was to let the work speak for itself knowing that the proof lies in the eating of the pudding. I learned that such an approach is dangerous because we don't eat the pudding for a long time; and the instant expert will have long gone on his merry way, leaving a trail of wreckage behind. I have developed very firm convictions that we need to be able to stand on our own two feet and defend our judgment and ourselves in a public arena. There is nothing more unequal than a banner headline about an instant critic on the front page on one day, and a little square on the back page two days later . . . on behalf of the maligned accused. The more violent the statement, the bigger the headline. The bigger the subject, the more it is quoted the next time around.

Newspapers are out to sell papers, and headlines are what sell papers. They will give you equal space if you are able to stand up and contest for it. But they are not going to do your work for you, and they are not going to hold the presses while you get ready. There are, of course, in the public all degrees of knowledge and sophistication and your answers will have to reach them all.

Some time ago I happened to be at a certain midwest airport when a pilot called in to ask the time. The tower asked who he was. The pilot answered, "What difference does it make? I want to know the time of the day!" The tower then answered, "Well— if you're Pan-Am, it's 1400 hours; if you're United, it's 2:00

o'clock; and if you are Ozark Airlines, the little hand is on the two and the big hand is straight up."

There will be many tens of millions of dollars spent during our lifetime in the name of environment. If we are knowledgeable, intelligent, and have a good dialogue with the public, these dollars will be spent wisely. If we are not intelligently informed and communicate poorly with the public, many billions of these dollars will be spent on ill-conceived projects and programs carried forward under public pressure that we did not foresee and did not intelligently work with.

FIFTH, LET'S TALK ABOUT OUR NEW GENERATION. The more quoted sound and fury, the more the young generation believes that the older generation—or the establishment—has done it again. The younger generation is our public and is growing in importance. Its sheer weight of numbers bears this out. By 1980, it is projected that there will be forty-eight million youths in the eighteen to thirty age group and that this group will constitute thirty percent of the voting population. These students are our next generation, and we must effectively bring them into the productive fold. We must also realize that they will not come as a monolithic generation of new graduates. They will come in with a much broader education, and sharp awareness of the social sciences, the humanities, and of the environment.

And it is not just the young but a wider spectrum of people who are interested in the environment. Here is a quotation which I just happened to see a few months ago in the *Saturday Review*. "Why these corporations are so short-sighted in this important public relations field, I cannot understand, but instead of volunteering to join in smog abatement, they are resisting it. I have just about reached the conclusion that, while large industry is important, fresh air and clean water are more important; and the day will come when we have to lay that kind of a hand on the table and see who is bluffing." Now who do you think said that? That was Senator Barry Goldwater, who is hardly the liberal long-haired type. So we see that concern for the environment is not the private preserve of youth, or the ultra-liberal.

LAST, LET US VISUALIZE OUR CITIES FROM OUR OWN PERSPECTIVE.

FOR EXAMPLE, AS A PHYSICIAN MIGHT LOOK AT A HUMAN BODY WITH ALL ITS LIFE SYSTEMS. The *metabolic system* is the network which provides for the ingestion, each day, each minute of each day, each second of each minute, of huge quantities of waters, supplies, air, food, and fuel and the consequent production of natural waste. I am talking here of the fantastic machine—*nature*. Nature, like the human body, is an ever-changing network when totally left alone. Nature made our canyons, our mesas, our plains. Nature changes itself more so than any futile human being could ever do. The judicious addition of reservoirs, dams, power plants, communities, and sewage treatment plants is only a part, and minute at that, added to the overwhelming natural metabolic system.

The *cardio-vascular system* or the horizontal and vertical paths of movement, and objects which move along them like boats on lakes, tracks and trains, highways and automobiles, stairways and people. While the veins and arteries themselves are static, as in the human body, the movement of objects and people along these pathways is dynamic (like a blood stream).

The *nervous system* or the information communication network of the environment which makes it possible for any of its many parts to keep in touch and be managed as an entity: telephone switching centers, electrical distribution networks, TV, traffic control signals, street signs; all are part of this nervous system allowing the community to survive, like the brain and nervous system of a man.

The *enclosure or three-dimensional system* is the combination of natural and man-made structures that surround the hollow places of the area in which the life of the community goes on. We must think in terms of an aesthetic system, like the beauty of the human body. The word *aesthetic* in French means *watch out!!* I am proposing to settle for a sort of reserved approach and state that those of us responsible for the erection of three-dimensional objects should not do anything willfully ugly or offensive. This, of course, leaves lots of room for all kinds of things that people might think are nice or terrible. This is far from meaning that there should not be discussion or emotional arguments over what is good or bad aesthetically. Quite the contrary. The things that I personally believe should not be implemented are those things that nobody objects to.

Our environment, our man-made structure, looks different in the winter, in the summer, in the rain, in the sunshine. It looks different under a clear blue sky, or reflected into a magnificent clouded day. Our environment looks different to a fisherman on the shore, to a hunter in the hills, to an Indian in the plains. Our environment will look different to passengers in an automobile travelling sixty miles per hour on our highways, to a bicycle rider, or to a walking pedestrian tourist gazing at nature (or at girls). Our environment will look different to a businessman in the air, flying from coast to coast. It will look different through a window from a house. It will look different to a worker in a plant. There are a myriad of perceptive levels that an environmental designer must consider.

AND FINALLY, WE MUST HAVE A FEELING FOR PEOPLE. With our present capacity for problem-solving, we do our most spectacular work when there is little or no social context. We are more skilled in coping with problems not involving the human factor. But there has never been a complete physical plant having no relevance to some social conditions. We build new highways because people need them; we need new businesses and medical complexes because our society needs facilities where economic trends or health needs can be met. We are constantly translating social needs into physical forms.

We cannot afford the luxury of ignoring the impact of rapid social change, urbanization, technological development, the need for new schools, new hospitals, new educational and medical systems, libraries and museums. We cannot afford to ignore the immediate issues of our society: old age, retirement years, shorter working hours, and more leisure time. We cannot ignore the fact that over eighty percent of our American families cannot afford to buy a new home.

Be it an oil well, a hospital, an industrial park, a whole city, the planning of the entire state or a single building, these facilities are all built by people for people. The need for environmental beauty, like the need for clean air, the need to see a tree, or a clear stream of water, is as basic to man as the need for food, work, and housing. If this need is not satisfied, man gradually sinks into frustration and ineffectiveness.

There is more to our culture, our society, our professions, than return on investment, price per visit, profit per manhour, smoke and noise abatement, industrial parks, and never-empty or never-ending roads. There are people, fields, trees, museums, theaters, hospitals, and libraries. Most of all there are people—people with ideals, prejudices, love—people who dream and procrastinate, sleep and accomplish, people who are angry, peaceful, driving and complacent. These people are our opportunity and our future.

Chapter 5

THE CHURCH AS A THERAPEUTIC COMMUNITY

REV. DAN R. KENNEDY

Religion and Community Mental Health

IN 1961, when the Joint Commission on Mental Illness and Health published their final report, *Action for Mental Health,* they indicated that forty-two percent of the persons who encounter mental or emotional distress seek out the assistance of a clergyman as the first person to whom they turn for help.[1] Since that time there has been a rapid acceleration of the recognition of the possible roles of the clergy in the total mental health program of a community.

However, the religious leader probably does more for the total mental health of a community by the care and nurture of his own religious community. Wider community recognition does not change the importance of the nature of the internal emotional life of a religious community. I believe the voluntary religious community can be a practicum for meeting the crises of life for some eighty million Americans who consider themselves part of an organized religious body. These persons can then potentially affect the mental health of the larger community outside the church, locally and nationally.

A Model Religious Community

The University Church of Goleta, United Methodist, has attempted to achieve self-consciousness as a therapeutic community. This church has a year round membership of about 150 persons who live in the student community of Isla Vista and the nearby Goleta Valley. Located near the University of California at Santa Barbara, the church attracts over 3,000 students each year into some aspect of its program and involves over 400 young adults into some type of face-to-face activity or group.

101

One image of a religious therapeutic community which needs to be overcome is described by Peter de Vries in his book, *The Mackarel Plaza,* which pictures *Peoples Liberal* as:

> the first split level church in America. It has a Neuro-psychiatric wing that is indefinitely expandable. The church interior is convertible into an auditorium for putting on plays, a gymnasium for athletics, and a ballroom for dances. There is a small worship area at one end. The liberalized hymnal has such masterworks of devotion as "Has Anyone Seen Kelly?" The pulpit consists of a slab of marble set on four legs of delicately differing fruit woods, to symbolize the four gospels and their failure to harmonize. Rev. Mackarels' last sermon was on the theme, "It is the final proof of God's omnipotence, that he need not exist in order to save us."[2]

I do not believe a church becomes a therapeutic community merely by professionalizing or striving to meet a psycho-social norm. Rather, by staying within its self-defined religious task and by being authentic to its own identity, it has its best chance to become therapeutic. Thus, the worship area needs to remain central and not become *a small area at one end.*

Therapeutic Worship

The religious community affirms worship as a central task of its existence. If a religious community is seeking health in its interpersonal relationships, one should be able to find a therapeutic dimension in the worship practice.

Worship is the ritualistic core of the community's mythology. It is at the center of the *inbreathing* of the community. All the other activities of the community ebb and flow in relationship to the nature of the worship. Hopefully it is the time when the church comes together to focus its mythological identity, and when the people are able to make themselves present to each other. Worship is the symbolic reliving of the heritage of the community, the empowering for its future, and the key to fulfilling its present moment.

Too often the church fails by not taking itself seriously enough. It finds the world's crisis and its own existence too hard to handle and slips off into the alienated imagination of Freud's *Illusion* and Marx's *Opiate.* Worship is the time when the authority dynamic in the community surfaces, and the time when the church can deal with its authenticity or nonauthenticity. The first task of worship as a therapeutic practice is to deal with its own nonbeing and the patterns of nonbeing within the worshipping community.

Classic Resistance

The cutting edge of growth in the therapeutic community is not creativity and innovation, but the encountering of its own resistance patterns to change and authority. Recognizing the nature of resistance during the worship hour and dealing with the patterns of transference is the classic definition of the therapeutic task in worship. Wilhelm Reich's definition of resistance in the therapeutic hour applies also to the patterns of resistance found in people's attitudes, actions, and feelings during the worship hour.[3]

Reich believed that the resistance encountered during the therapeutic hour related to the same patterns of resistance found in the client's life outside the therapeutic hour. The resistance found in the worship hour would relate to the same type of resistance pattern found in the life stance of the worshiper outside the worship hour. A listless hymn can be listened to with the same degree of insight as the listless voice of the client during a therapeutic encounter. The worshiper will avoid awareness, displace responsibility, maintain his personal or group alienation, and protect his loneliness during the worship experience in the same way he maintains his inauthentic relationship to the rest of his life. Since worship is one of man's deepest rituals by which he can learn to love, to maintain prejudices, or even to encounter his whole self, the worship experience can be the very source and process of the worshiper's nonbeing.

Institutional and environmental resistance peculiar to the religious community can be overwhelming. In protestant Christianity some of the institutional resistance relates to preconceived ideas about the meaning of the worship hour, the nature of the sermon, the place of authority of the minister, and the nature of the preacher's and the liturgist's task.

The Pew

The greatest environmental enemy to the emotional health of church worship is the pew! The pew has become one of the architectural necessities of sanctuary construction. It is an indicator of people's expectations of themselves when they worship. The pew implies that the worshiper can just sit quietly and let God take care of everything through the *mana* of the minister and the choir. This pattern translated into everyday life implies that the *responsible* person can just sit quietly through life and let those outside of himself make the decisions and do all the work.

No matter what the minister says about responsible action, or how well the choir sings the anthem, the worshiper will have received support for a depressive and inactive life style because he sits quietly in the wooden straight jacket called the pew. The pew is symbolic of the killing of personal responsibility and individual action.

Inaction within the worshipping community relates to inaction outside of the church community. What is at stake in the worship of a therapeutic religious community is the nature of its actions, or in theological language, the dimensions of its Sacramental Life.

The University Church of Goleta worship service has emphasized movement and action in all parts of the worship.[4] There are no pews, thus seating and movement has open-ended possibilities. People are provided opportunities to participate in all aspects of the service. During the singing, everybody sings; during the sacramental celebration itself, everybody is given the opportunity to move around and participate, even to dance if the person so desires. During the sermon opportunities for involvement are provided. Instead of one man talking, everybody participates and all persons are given the task of putting content into the worship experience.

The Communal Sermon

The communal sermon is a theological effort to bring meaningful action, i.e. the Sacrament, into the presentation of cognitive material, i.e. the Word. It is an action variant on the monologue presentation. In the communal service, people participate in the experiencing of ideas and create the sermon for themselves. The minister becomes a catalyst for group activity and participation. During the communal sermon persons interact with other persons in groups of six or eight. They play with blocks, color with crayons, or use some other simple tool of expression in order to wrestle with theological ideas and to experience them in relation to other persons. They function in a context that encourages them to take themselves seriously.

The communal sermon as a catalyst to encounter rather than a package of truth, can open the possibility of discovering the individual self as incomplete, perhaps absurd, and human. This self-view can bring about a recovery of authentic dealing with a person's secret feelings of guilt and shame.

The questions of Genesis 3:9-13 do not have *right* answers, but in the context of the communal sermon they can lead to individual experiential responses. The detailed questioning of *What, Where, and How* can bring authenticity to the worshiper's own existence. Adam's flight is the mythological resistance pattern to which the questions are addressed. His problem is to face the feelings and reality of his own existence. The worshiper's task is to accept feelings about his own existence.

At the depth of the Biblical *Mythical History* the dynamics of the *Why* of life are explored by the questions of *Where, What, and How*. The monologue sermon, which thoroughly explains the why of life by dealing only on the cognitive level, misses the opportunity for detailing the active interaction which is possible through *Where, What and How*. This interaction is what the communal sermon attempts to provide.

Therapeutic Values of the Communal Sermon
Floating

Floating is a nonstructured time during the communal sermon when groups and individuals are seeking self-definition. When a group begins an exercise there is an uncomfortable time before any direction for the group comes into focus. These are very important moments when the fears and desires of the individual become present for utilization. Floating is a normal part of everyday existence. Everything we encounter in life does not come ready-packaged with the decision process already easily defined.

Many people come to worship to escape this type of everyday pressure and miss the type of self-affirmation creative floating invites. However, church during worship is considered a safe place by most people. Quite often they will risk more in church than in any other circumstance. Many people feel protected in church and will participate in activities of higher personal vulnerability than in everyday life. One morning a man came up after church and said he found the experience quite frightening. He explained he was in therapy, and that if this had happened in any other place he would have had to run out. However, since he was in church, he decided nothing could happen to him and he would try to stick it out.

At the start of the communal sermon directions are given, but it is up to the individual to respond. Quite often there are seconds, and even minutes, when people in a small circle will just look at each other. The tense situation which yet is safe, as in floating, will accustom people to get involved more readily and to know how to find their own level of motivation in tough everyday situations.

Feedback

There is little opportunity for feedback in the monologue sermon. There is only very limited chance for the minister to discover if he has communicated during his statement. The only morning the preacher knows where he stands is when he makes people angry, and they find new doors out of the church rather than have to shake his hand.

The communal sermon is a place of interaction. A person will have many opportunities to see how he functions in many different situations. He will be able to see how his functioning relates to his own statements of value and faith, and to the statements of values and faith of other persons.

In one of the communal sermon groups a woman who was in church for the first time was able to talk to strangers about the loss of her husband. This was the first time she had been able to share her sorrow and the fear of being left alone and growing old by herself. Her group was very supportive, and she received a strong *feedback* of care and concern.

> Sue was always nervous during her group in church. When the time to share verbally came, she would immediately begin talking and monopolize the entire time. For several weeks she was the only person in her group to talk. Finally, one Sunday, Margaret could stand it no longer and broke into what Sue was saying with a very loud and angry, "Damn it, shut up!" Sue stopped in surprise and then began crying. She confessed she was afraid of what would happen in the group if she did not "make it happen." She instead controlled the group by not allowing any silence. She got plenty of comments as to how the group had seen her, much of it given in a relatively unaggressive manner, and she and Margaret were still talking long after the worship was over.[5]

Feedback from persons we trust is an important way in which people understand themselves and learn to perceive the motivation of their behavior.

Healing

The church community is a place where people can experience situations in which they can be caring and loving people. They also can encounter their own lives at occasions when they need love, and realize that they are capable of receiving love and care from persons.

One of the *tenets* of the church is that one *should* be loving and take care of people in need. This ideal is presented quite often, but usually no help is given in understanding *how* to be a loving and caring person. Many people have experienced the frustration of trying to be a *do-gooder* but have no experience in helping.

The worship setting can provide the practicum for a person to learn to see himself as a loving and caring person. At the University Church of Goleta one form of communal prayer is used to help people get in touch with each other. People gather together in groups of three and four. The minister leads a meditation in which he first helps people to become aware of themselves by asking a series of questions followed by pauses. Can they become aware of their feet on the floor? How are they sitting?

How does their breathing feel to them? Then, in the time of quiet which follows, a theme to focus on in a personal way is presented, and the people are given a short time to think about this idea or experience. Then, using the symbols of the community, the people are invited to reach out and physically encounter the other people in the group. Saying the words "Where two or three are gathered together in my name, there I am also," the minister asks the people to share the content of the meditation with others in the group. Permission is always given not to share if someone does not wish to reveal the content of his meditative excursion.

> June, her husband Frank, and Carol were sitting in a group. June and Carol had had a disagreement during the week over church finances that had not been resolved. The meditative task was to remember a time in their lives when they had been lonely.
>
> Carol began by sharing an incident when she had been very ill and had committed herself to the mental hospital in Camarillo, California. She described being locked in a ward and she began to cry. June took her hand and held it while she talked and cried. As Carol stopped June self-consciously pulled her hand back, but Carol would not let go and said, "No, no, keep it there. I like that."
>
> Then June began to share her meditation on her own loneliness which was a time she was in the hospital for the birth of one of her sons. She knew the Rh factor was not right and there had to be a blood transfusion. The nurse came into the room and, as she laid out the dress clothes June had brought to take the baby home in, she said that if they had a priest or minister he should be called right away. Her son was in very critical condition, but June mistakenly thought the nurse was implying that he had died. With the telling of the experience June began to cry. The two ladies hugged each other tightly and cried together for a while.
>
> Frank then said, "I don't have anything to share that will match you ladies. When I was a freshman in college, having left home in Idaho to attend USC, I found myself alone in Los Angeles over the Christmas vacation. All of my friends had left and I had received no note or gift from my parents. It was a lonely, lonely time for me. I feel outdone by you ladies though, because I can't really cry about my story."
>
> The first lady, Carol, was still crying and had exhausted her supply of Kleenex, so Frank reached into his back pocket and pulled out a large red and blue bandana type of kerchief. As he handed it to her she couldn't help but laugh, and she said, "Oh, Frank, I love you for that," and with that Frank began to cry and they all held onto each other.[6]

These three people were in their late thirties and had all the middle class reserve about holding one's composure in public. I do believe that they risked a lot during the sharing, but they also experienced themselves as warm and loving people. They shared a need and experienced that they could expose themselves and be taken care of, and that they were capable of taking care of another person.

Conflict

Even though religious groups proclaim themselves agents of reconciliation, they seldom deal successfully with conflict within the congregation or even outside in the community. Usually conflict is avoided, and in the context of worship conflict is *prayed for* but otherwise kept at arm's distance. Direct confrontation with a social issue offends many church people who come to worship to *escape* the concerns of the world.

The communal sermon gives a great opportunity to approach a *touchy* subject in a context different from the lecture sermon, which usually just raises the level of the prejudice or hostility on a particular issue. On Vietnam, as on any item of social concern, a great deal of tension is evident in the congregation as the subject is approached. The opportunity to air feelings and to discuss the problem in an authentic fashion is simply not present during a monologue sermon. My experience of dealing with Vietnam is one of frustration in the structure of the *straight* monologue sermon. Because there is no opportunity for encounter, people leave under such a high load of anger, usually directed at the preacher, that only the bravest of men would attempt to deal with such bottled-up emotions.

In the communal sermon Vietnam was dealt with in a role-playing situation. Slips of paper were prepared by members of the Political Science Department of the University of California at Santa Barbara which laid out the positions of the United States, of the Saigon Government, of the Viet Cong, of North Vietnam, of the Red Chinese, of Russia, of the National Liberation Front, and of Pope Paul. (Pope Paul of course in reality would not be there, but we wanted some figure to represent the futility of being the church in the situation.) As the groups formed, these slips of paper were given out randomly to each person. They were to visualize themselves as coming to a peace table. The slip of paper told them who they represented and what the attitudes of that role were to be.

Before the slips could be handed out a debate started in one of the groups between a *dove* and a *hawk*. When they got the slips, they happened to receive a position completely opposite to their own personal belief. They participated with their roles reversed. Afterwards they both confessed that they had to look at the validity of the arguments of the other side for the first time. As the service ended there were many discussions between the people over the issue, and the level of tension was not high.

A simulation game was used to deal with the race problem. The whole service was a role playing incident. The sanctuary was divided into four sections of town: *Dead End Flats*, the slum of the city, with no chairs; *West Side*, with wooden chairs very tightly compacted; *Paradise Garden*, with metal chairs and some plants and space; and *Mount Olympus*, with leather chairs, potted plants, coffee and cookies.

A very involved ethnic breakdown with a number of tension points was designed into the situation, the most pressing being the lack of chairs in the crowded slum section. During the morning the slum section revolted, yelling "We want chairs" and running to the part of the city where chairs were available. Wrestling for chairs occurred all over the sanctuary. After the revolt a City Council meeting was called to discuss the problem, each section of town appointing one speaker. The speakers were picked by a variety of means in each part of town, mob rule in Dead End Flats and a variety of democratic processes in the other sections. The City Council met with picketing and protest songs, etc., from Dead End Flats.

In the process of the game both individual and group conflict was experienced. During the revolt there were real screams of fear and tears of anger as people fought over chairs. Two liberals from Mount Olympus later tried to give their chairs to people from Dead End Flats and were hooted down with calls of *tokenism*.

The groups broke into mixed discussion after the *game* and

had more to work with in terms of feelings than was possible to deal with in the time remaining. Talk continued long after the morning service was over.

The change of attitude and growth toward openness during these two experiences was measurable. This type of opportunity to deal with conflict is not present in the straight sermon context.

A girl came up to me afterwards. She was living in Mt. Olympus during the simulation and was in tears because she had never done anything like *that* in her life. This boy had come up and wanted her chair, so they had fought, and she had swung and hit him. She wanted to talk about her feelings during the service.

Simulation and role playing are simple educational tools. Applying them in a worship context opens "hot" areas of human concern to reconciliation.

Ecce Homo

Perhaps the church provides the most therapeutic context when it is least preoccupied with its own fellowship and most strenuously losing its life in its servant task in the world.

On February 26, 1970 the Isla Vista branch of the Bank of America was burned and the neighborhood of the Isla Vista church changed to an area torn by violence. The normal meetings of the church ceased and many groups, including the worship committee, met on the street while they were trying to keep community peace. They talked about the context of worship in the *Do-nut Shop* rather than in the meeting rooms of the church. The church moved its center of action into the community with organized direction. Individuals in the church took on community responsibility. The coordinator of the Community Activities Board was a student member of the church. The Speakers Bureau at the University was run by a student from our church. The president of the Isla Vista Association was a member of the church.

A time of extreme crisis occurred when the university refused Jerry Rubin the opportunity to speak on campus. The church was asked if he could speak on its property. The Administrative Board met for some eight hours over a period of four days trying to keep peace in Isla Vista. The problem was, as they saw it, that an easy *yes* would not lower the possibilities of peace, nor would a hard *no*, which might lead to reprisals. They searched to find a way to defuse the situation and let the man speak in the community and keep free speech alive.

After several hours of discussion they directed the ministers to gather together the widest possible representation of the leadership of Isla Vista to see if some community-wide decision could be reached. The sheriff, members of the administration of the university, merchants, property owners, landlords, radicals, and student leaders met for a day to try to arrive at a mutually agreeable plan. They arrived at a plan which they could all support and which had a low risk of violence. They took the plan to the County Board of Supervisors and received a unanimous turndown on the public permit. The hard no had been delivered. The week following was one of Isla Vista's most violent, ending in death for Kevin Moran, a student. This was a sad, frustrating time for the people of the church. They had come close to a solution of conflict, but they had failed.

The levels of trust and confidence that had developed between people during worship experiences was the glue which held them together during this trying time. Some church members moved to support views differing from their own prejudgments because they trusted the other church members whom they knew to be closer to the situation and able to make more valid decisions. Members who lived outside of Isla Vista withheld judgment and left the decisions to the people living in Isla Vista who could more realistically access the situation. The church experience in Berkeley, California, during its time of violence showed most churches there split wide open because of the differing attitudes of members who lived in Berkeley and of those who lived outside the city. Intimate encounter during worship experiences had built a high level of trust and confidence in our congregation which let the church unify its strength so that it could deal with the community disruption.

During the week of violence in Isla Vista many members, both student and adult, had their backs against the walls of the temporary Bank of America trying to protect the building and to maintain the community as a place where persons could live in peace. The chairman of the worship committee wrestled a ladder away from a man trying to get on the roof. Members on the bank's front porch asked rioters why they were throwing rocks and every so often offered therapeutic blows themselves. I am not sure of the actual therapeutic value of much of this violent activity, but it was individual action on the part of church members which kept overt violence, for awhile, from exploding in Isla Vista.

The vitality with which the church moved out of its internal institutional functioning into the larger community was related to the trust the members had established with each other over several years of encounters during communal forms of sermon and prayer. The therapeutic religious community offers a continual experience of self and community not obtainable by the isolated week-end experience at Esalen and Kairos. The growth and experience of the Self within a communal continuum generates a momentum which produces responsible people in times of civic disruption.

The communal sermon is a hybrid of communication techniques and personal sensitivity. I believe it forms a context that can, in theological terms, lead to a mythological nowness where the person is free to understand himself as a creative and loving person.

In 1920, Thornton Wilder wrote a one-act play called, "The Angel Who Troubled the Waters." The following lines of the play apply to the self-image that members of The University Church of Goleta have of themselves. The play is based on the fifth chapter of the Gospel of John where an angel comes to the pool of Bethesda and troubles the waters. It is said that the first person entering the waters will be healed.

In the play a physician goes to Bethesda to be healed. He would have been the first to immerse himself in the water but the angel stops him and says, "Draw back physician, this moment is not for you." And the physician says, "Angelic visitor, I pray thee, listen to my prayer." And the angel, "Healing is not for you." The physician, "Surely the angels are wise, surely, Oh Prince, you are not deceived by my apparent wholeness. Your eyes can see the nets in which my wings are caught, the sin into which all my endeavors sink half-performed cannot be concealed from you." And the angel says, "I know." Physician: "Oh, in such an hour was I born and doubly fearful to me is the flaw in my heart. Must I drag my shame, Prince and Singer, all the days more bowed than my neighbor?" Angel: "Without your wound, where would your power be? It is your very remorse that makes your low voice tremble into the hearts of men. The very angels themselves cannot persuade the wretched and blundering children on earth as can one human being broken on the wheels of living. In love's service only the wounded soldier can serve—draw back."

The person who was the first into the pool was healed, came up, and said to the physician, "Come with me to my house; my son is lost in dark thoughts. I do not understand him, and only you have ever lifted his mood. And my daughter, by the hour sits, since her child has died, in the shadow; she will not listen to us."[7]

Care more than emphasis on cure, and understanding and acceptance more than adjustment, are the most important words in the religious therapeutic community. The religious therapeutic community consists of those people who have climbed the forbidden tree, eaten the forbidden fruit, and yet come down in a new state of grace. The therapeutic church community dares to join hands with Jacob of Old and wrestle with life and with God for the sacramental potential of humanness. Then with a new understanding and acceptance of what whole broken humanness means, limps with Jacob into the future.

BIBLIOGRAPHY

1. Joint Commission on Mental Illness and Health: *Action for Mental Health*. New York, Basic Books, 1961.
2. De Vries, Peter: *The Mackarel Plaza*. Boston, Little, Brown and Co., 1958, p. 13.
3. Reich, Wilhelm: *Character Analysis*. New York, Farrar, Straus and Giroux, Inc., 1949.
4. University Church of Goleta offers two worship modes each week. The communal sermon is part of the celebrative or *Dionysian* experiential service. A second *Apollonian* approach is presented in a more meditative mode at a different time.
5. Kennedy, Dan: Personal Notes. Spring, 1968.
6. Kennedy: *op. cit.*, Fall, 1968.
7. Wilder, Thornton: *The Angel That Troubled the Waters and Other Plays*. New York, Coward-McCann, 1928, p. 147ff.

Chapter 6

DEMOCRATIC INSTITUTIONS AND MENTAL HEALTH

FRANK K. KELLY

IN THE INTRODUCTION to this program, some important statements were made: "Never in the history of man has an individual had at the same time so much and so little freedom. . . . War and racism and poverty run rampant in our cities and world communities. Essential to the solution of all these people problems is the understanding of man's psychological and social nature and the development of practical and effective remedial action."

Where can one take hold of these enormous problems? It may be evidence of insanity to contend that anyone can understand the relationships between democratic institutions and mental health. At the Center where I work, we have suspected ourselves of megalomania and mental gluttony but we go on racing from question to question, hoping to see the connections, trying to get our fellow citizens to think in different ways, feeling that mankind cannot be abandoned to the tidal waves of confusion that boom and crash more loudly and more rapidly every day.

Shuddering from the task of preparing this paper, wondering why I was so ready to bite off more than I can chew, I found myself sustained by the bravery of Dr. Joshua Bierer. Dr. Carleton sent me a copy of a book, *Innovations in Social Psychiatry*, containing dialogues between Dr. Bierer and Dr. Evans.

I found Dr. Bierer saying: "The more we progress technologically, the more we regress in understanding and handling each other as groups and as individuals. . . ." This is a phenomenon which has engaged us at the Center for some years. The machines that serve us appear to be destroying us. How can we change our institutions to cope with the machines? Can man's mind and spirit stretch to cope with the awareness of swift and endless change?

I also found Dr. Bierer saying:

It might appear that we are progressing. For example, communication has been made so much easier. In one second, the whole
world can know something. The President of the United States,
John Kennedy, was assassinated; the next instant the whole world
knew about it. However, the world does not realize that only in
the case of sensational events has communication been facilitated.
In the field of science, communication is much slower, one of the
obvious reasons being that science has developed to such a degree
that it is impossible for any one person to cover the entire field. As
an editor, I find that the majority of writers from America have no
idea what happens in Britain, and vice versa. In fact, they are
two different worlds, even though the British and the Americans
seem to speak the same language.

The implications in these statements of Dr. Bierer could lead
one into despair. Our technology has made it possible for us
to destroy one another—and all the life around us. But we have
not learned how to understand one another, to accept each
other, to help one another effectively even though we now know
that our failures in human relations may destroy this beautiful
world.

But Dr. Bierer has not fallen into despair. He has gone on
thinking, working, experimenting. Using his own freedom to
choose hope, he has brought hope to many frightened and tor-
mented people. Out of the many ideas about the nature of man
available to him, he has chosen a view of man as a being with
many capacities for growth. He has devised day hospitals and
therapeutic communities in his efforts to "reduce the tremendous waste of human energy, suffering, and money to a minimum."

At the Center, we have often been tempted to despair. We have
heard all the prophets of doom. We have been confronted by the
inertia and apathy that afflict so many people. We have been
threatened with personal attacks and rumors of bombs. We have
been subjected to the wild suspicions of right-wing extremists
and the scorn of young radicals who regard our devotion to reason
as a relic of a vanished age.

This has been called a Time of Troubles, a Crisis of Crises, an
Age of Aquarius. It might be more accurately called a Period of

Paranoia. Anxieties breed distrust and distrust produces anxieties and the Circles of Fear grow wider and wider.

We are often told these days that man is a tool-making animal, an aggressive animal, a territorial animal, a naked ape, a bio-mechanical link, a crossing point where cosmic radiation and electromagnetic fields shape and swing atoms and molecules. We are seldom reminded that man can also be regarded as a rational being.

Believers in democracy choose to believe that man has a mysterious and marvelous mind; not simply a brain, which can be described as a very cunning computer, but a mind, a power that uses a brain for purposes beyond those of a computer. This mind can be blocked from development to its full height and breadth and depth. This mind can be choked by fear, deceived by passion, distracted by a torrent of sensations but it can also be an arrow of light, cutting through confusion, illuminating what human beings are supposed to be.

With such beliefs, we act on assumptions that cannot be bolstered by completely convincing demonstrations. We assume that people have a certain wisdom which can be guided and developed. We assume that people need leaders but often stride ahead of those leaders. We assume that machines created by man can be controlled by man. We assume that communications can be improved and even the English and the Americans will learn to understand one another.

I think there is evidence to indicate that democratic institutions and mental health are closely related. People in the countries with such institutions came through World War II with more confidence in the future than people in the totalitarian countries. People in the freer countries face up to the burdens of guilt more openly in many cases than those who have submitted to dictatorships.

We are all guilty in many ways. As we recognize our common guilt, we begin to share responsibility for humanity. The sharing of this responsibility is essential to the democratic process. We can make democracy work, if we can engage in effective two-way communication, listening freely as well as speaking freely.

In order to do any of the tremendously difficult things we must do to build a really free and really just society, we must have confidence in the future. A sign of mental health is a willingness to face the future without dread, without being overcome by the threatening storms that converge upon us. We cannot rely upon chemical tranquilizers. We cannot blur the sharp edges of enormous problems with alcohol or any of the easy remedies offered to us.

At the Center, we have recently proposed a broad context for consideration of the basic issues confronting our society. We have offered the people a model constitution designed to meet the needs of the turbulent times in which we live.

The preamble to the Constitution of 1787 lists six objectives:

> We the people of the United States, in order to form a more perfect union, establish justice, insure domestic tranquillity, provide for the common defense, promote the general welfare, and secure the blessings of liberty to ourselves and our posterity do ordain and establish this Constitution. . . .

The preamble to the proposed model constitution cites three goals:

> So that we may join in common endeavors, welcome the future in good order, and create an adequate and self-repairing government —we the people do establish the United Republics of America, herein provided to be ours, and do ordain this Constitution, whose law it shall be until the time provided for it shall have run.

Note the emphasis on welcoming the future in good order. The spirit of hope for humanity and confidence in man's capacity breathes through those words.

Can we have a realistic hope that man does have a future? I think we can. Looking at the history of this nation and the history of mankind we can be appalled by the wars and the waste of millions of lives, or we can be astonished by the persistence of man's search for better ways. We can see that man can be a destructive monster or creature, striving to awaken from the ancient nightmares of blood and vengeance, striving to become a being shaped in the image and likeness of a noble idea; the idea of a loving, creative God.

Man trembles on the brink of self-annihilation. Trembling, he stops to think. Thinking, he knows he must plan for the future. Planning, he develops more flexible institutions in which every one finds more open paths of participation. Participating and co-operating, he learns what it means to be a whole person. To be whole is to be holy, to be healthy in mind and body, to awake and sing.

Welcome the future in good order. Know what self-government calls for. Build a self-repairing government. These are the things we must do. If we can think of them, we can do them.

In the proposed constitution, "we the people" has a much broader scope than "we the people" did in 1787. In those days, each slave was counted as "three-fifths" of a person. Women could not vote. Power was firmly in the hands of a small number of property owners.

In 1971, "we the people" means everybody. The 18-year-olds were recently given the right to vote for federal officials, and some states are extending that right to include participation in all elections. Young people of all ages now make their views known and those views have to be considered in the new planning that is needed at every level.

In 1971, everybody is becoming very conscious of the runaway technology to which Dr. Bierer referred. The facts of life are brought home to all of us when we see the pollution in the air, when we know there may be poison in our food, when we gag upon the stench of polluted lakes and rivers, when we find that the oceans are spotted with garbage. We no longer accept the excuses of the industrialists or the procrastination of politicians. We know that old ways and old delays will not save our planet.

In the new constitution, there is a reminder of citizens' duties as well as rights. People are expected to participate in a continuous discussion of public issues, and the government is expected to maintain a peaceful atmosphere for such discussions. Nothing is to be regarded as too controversial for full examination in public meetings. Such gatherings are to be protected against disruption. The new constitution assumes that we must devote as much time to participation in government through discussion as we now give to football, prize-fighting and baseball.

Planning, properly understood, is at the heart of the democratic system. The new constitution provides for three new branches of government; a planning branch, an electoral branch, and a regulatory branch. The planning branch would be organized to encourage the highest degree of citizen participation. The national planning board would offer outlines of steps to be taken over a twelve-year period and a six-year period; but these outlines would be implemented one year at a time. At public hearings, specific criticisms of each step would be invited.

One section of the proposal for a Planning Branch relates the nation to the rest of the world. Section 13 says: "In making plans, there shall be due regard to the interests of other nations and such cooperation with their intentions as may be consistent with the plans for the United Republics of America."

In the part of Article V dealing with the new House of Representatives, there are several statements about the international responsibilities of the House:

"To assist in the maintenance of world order, and for this purpose, when the President shall recommend, to vest such jurisdiction in international legislative, judicial or administrative organizations as shall be consistent with the national interest:

> To develop with other peoples, and for the benefit of all, the resources of space, of other bodies in the universe, and of the seas beyond twelve miles from low-water shores unless treaties shall provide other limits.
>
> To assist other peoples who have not attained satisfactory levels of well-being; to delegate the administration of funds, wherever possible, to international agencies; and to invest in or contribute to the furthering of development in other parts of the world.

In Article VIII—General Provisions—the model constitution declares in Section 15: "The President may make agreements with other organized peoples for a relation other than full membership in the United Republics. They may become citizens and may participate in the selection of officials. . . ."

Other countries could become Associated Republics. If their citizens voted to do so, they could share in the rights and responsibilities envisioned in this document, which has been designed for the twentieth century situation of mankind.

To open up such possibilities helps to bring the peoples of the world into friendlier relationships and such expanded democratic institutions can contribute to the mental health of humanity.

If the sane leaders of this planet are heeded, we may be on the verge of what Robert M. Hutchins has called *the learning society*. In his recent book bearing this title, he described it in these terms:

> This would be one that, in addition to offering part-time adult education to every man and woman at every stage of grown-up life, had succeeded in transforming its values in such a way that learning, fulfillment, becoming human, had become its aims and all its institutions were directed to this end.

I have focused much attention on the potentialities of a new constitution because I believe we can use this document to develop the new institutions we need so urgently. It offers us hope of coping with the problems which seem to have gone beyond our control.

Governor Rexford G. Tugwell, the principal author of the model constitution, worked for President Franklin D. Roosevelt, who once said: "The only thing we have to fear is fear itself."

With confidence in our ability to shape the future, we can cast away fear.

Death did not destroy the truth of what President John F. Kennedy once told us—we can bear any burden, meet any challenge we may have to face.

For those of us who believe in God, our confidence is based on the idea that man can praise God by affirming life and showing the creative and compassionate powers that come from a Being whose essence is love.

For those who believe primarily in man, there is evidence that man has tremendous insights; and man can change the world.

A year ago, I wrote an article for the *Saturday Review* on "The Possibilities of Transformation: A Report on the State of Mankind: 1970." I proposed the formation of a Council for Humanity, to give periodic reports on the directions in which humanity seemed to be moving. I received hundreds of letters from people in various countries who wanted to help in establishing such a council as a new democratic institution.

In the year since the publication of that article, I have noted some signs of transformation. The prospects for peace in the Middle East seem to be much greater: the people in Israel and the Arab countries have welcomed a long truce and are urging their governments to reach agreements. Although President Nixon's actions in Cambodia and Laos have discouraged many people, he keeps on insisting that he is *winding down* the Indo-China war. In fact, he said recently that there may never be another war!

Let us act upon these possibilities. Let us think together, pray together, and work together to help mankind to shake off the ultimate insanity—the insanity of war. Let us give thanks and praise to the Creative Power in the universe, the Power that pours through us when we open our minds and hearts to the people around us.

Let us welcome the future in good order!

Chapter 7

TRENDS IN CONTEMPORARY POLITICAL, SOCIAL AND CHURCH COMMUNITIES

PARTICIPANTS: Dr. C. H. Hardin Branch, moderator; Rev. Dan R. Kennedy, Frank Kelly, and Louis L. Rozenfeld

QUESTION: Mr. Kelly, in the development of our democratic system we have gotten rid of the hereditary sovereign. Would you say that we also did away with expecting the sovereign to do things for us? Do we, the people, have the attitudes necessary to operate a democratic society?

MR. KELLY: I don't think we have those attitudes among enough people. I think most people expect the system to work automatically or the so-called experts to solve every problem. If the experts make enough blunders, then people believe that they'll throw them out and get a new set. I don't think the people understand the concept of self-government. But as our educational level rises and as we get a higher percentage of people with good educational backgrounds, we have more and more of a chance to make democracy work.

QUESTION: Mr. Kelly, I have admired the work of the Center for the Study of Democratic Institutions for a long time. I've always found it a pity that it is not more publicized, and that the community is not drawn more into your wonderful work. How could this be done?

MR. KELLY: We did put on a series of five meetings at the Lobero Theater,* which were attended by hundreds of people. Our problem is that, in order to carry on the meetings at the Center (we have them four or five days a week), we have to bring together a group of people who focus on a particular problem. We can't spend a great deal of time explaining what we're doing. From time to time the local newspaper carries stories; in fact, they carried quite a few in recent months. People

---

* Santa Barbara.

still come up to me and say, "Why didn't I read about that in the paper?" It was in the paper! People are so busy that they can't absorb the information about the Center which is provided. We have seats open for observers at a lot of our meetings, and if anyone would like to attend the meeting, call me, as we try to schedule several weeks in advance.

QUESTION: Mr. Kelly, I have here a report of a national survey by the United States Office of Education, which brings into question the direction in which we are going. If I may read a few of these gruesome statistics: This was a survey of nine-, thirteen-, and seventeen-year-olds and young adults of ages twenty-six to thirty-five. The survey found that ninety-four percent of thirteen-year-olds, seventy-eight percent of seventeen-year-olds, and sixty-eight percent of young adults in this country voted in favor of censorship and against free speech. Eighty percent of nine-year-olds believe that the police have the right to enter anyone's home at any time. Half the thirteen-year-olds do not understand the basic right of peaceful assembly, and more than one third of thirteen- and seventeen-year-olds believe that the police should be able to monitor telephones. Now if this is the way the majority of today's American youth thinks, if they believe in an authoritarian order, we have set the stage for a fascist state. I'd welcome your comments, Mr. Kelly.

MR. KELLY: It looks that way, but I have become very skeptical of polls ever since I worked for Harry Truman in 1948. All my friends said, "Don't you know that Dewey is going to win by fourteen percent, or twenty-two percent?" Dewey had the elections sewed up, so Elmer Roper stopped polling in September. I don't think these kids were given these questions in a context which they fully understood. I also think there is a terrible deficiency in our schools, in that students are not taught about law and the whole process of self-government. That is why I have written my book, called *Your Laws*, which is aimed at young people. I was inspired to do this by Dr. Hutchins who said that teaching of the law, of the whole legal process, should begin in the grade school and shouldn't wait until high school when the student's ideas are already rigid.

QUESTION: Mr. Kelly, I don't think you really answered that

question. I know that what you say is true, I run a hot-line. People throw away their search-and-seizure rights and get into great difficulty. The tragedy of young people is their ignorance of the law. The schools are very quiet about this.

MR. KELLY: You're asking me to wrestle with the most difficult questions! It is hard to change curricula and introduce new courses. I've worked on the curriculum committee at Santa Barbara High School. We're trying to formulate a course on family and life, a so-called sex-education course. It's difficult for you run into so many bureaucratic procedures, or you find that you can't present it in a given way because the administrators wouldn't accept it. This whole process of approval has made our schools ineffective as educational instruments. You probably saw the recent report of the Carnegie commissions as well as that of the HEW task force which both stated that our present educational institutions are irrelevant to the basic needs of our society. This is one of the biggest problems we face and I haven't got all the answers.

QUESTION: Mr. Kelly, I would like your opinion on John Gardner's *Common Cause.*

MR. KELLY: I think John Gardner's *Common Cause* as an effort to set up a citizen's lobby is a good idea. I don't think it is a good idea to fragment our political parties more than they are. *Common Cause* is performing a good service and I hope it continues to expand. John Gardner can do what the Center cannot do, namely lobby. We at the Center provide ideas and thoughts; John Gardner and his people can take whatever ideas are useful and try to get them into legislative action.

DR. BRANCH: I would like to throw in a question of my own. Mr. Kennedy, it interests me that at the present time there seems to be a real renaissance of religious interest among young people of quite a *gut* quality; of the Pentecostal kind. I'm not enough in contact with it to be sure of my ground. It does seem to be a return to a primitive or highly emotional kind of religion, not an intellectual occupation with religious ideas. Do you care to make any comment, Dan, on why or if that is so?

REV. KENNEDY: I think this is so and I will refer to Reinhold Niebuhr on this, who said that when the day-to-day tasks become too tough men retreat into the absolute. Intellectually, the Jesus freaks are cop-outs but their enthusiasm is real. It was Santayana who said, "For man's religious life to take focus, it needs to appear to him in fantastic shapes."

The Jesus freaks express a need we should listen to. The liberal Protestant Church has become expert in psychology and sociology but it has failed to understand the dynamic of community, a dynamic which for a church is provided by a mythology, by a shared identity through Jesus Christ. The church has not concerned itself with this dynamic in a seriously intellectual endeavor, and therefore it's lost some steam.

Now what's happening with young people is a speeding up of a trend that always existed. UCSB* has some statistics on this. At times when emotional needs for a sense of community are not met by institutions, the liberal denominations always lose membership and the fundamentalist denominations gain. If the militant fundamentalist has a simple, compelling answer to a complex heart-rending personal problem, he convinces with his easy answer.

Part of the problem in our society is that the religious formulations concerning the relationship between soma and psyche have been neglected. Consequently many of the young people are not just going on the Jesus freak trip, but on a quest for answers from other esoteric, other more personal forms of religion, the Eastern religions or meditation. Basically they turn to formulations of religion that deal with concepts of self, loss of self in God and emergence of self from God. I believe that this is an authentic identity seeking. Many young people do it outside the church because they find that it is not being done to their satisfaction inside the church.

QUESTION: What you talk about seems to be growing rapidly on the campus. I've seen a large number of youths who first were on psychedelic drugs and then turned to the Pentecostal or other churches, or to transcendental meditation. Do you think there is a connection between the drug trips and the search into religions?

REV. KENNEDY: I feel there is a psychological connection be-

* University of California, Santa Barbara.

tween a Jesus freak trip and drug experimentation. The religious experience may be a more positively oriented loss of self but it doesn't really deal with the original problem. I think for some people it is life-saving and great. In terms of helping someone off a drug trip, I'd say that an intensely loving community will hold on to a person; the loving community really deals with the problem. (I've experienced this in moving people off heroin.) What goes on then is a community dynamic of people. They really take care of each other and focus on their personal identity within the theological community; this really grabs them.

DR. BRANCH: Louis, do you want to make a comment about this?

MR. ROZENFELD: We keep analyzing the symptom instead of talking about the cause of the disease. For thirty years now, I think, we have known that an overpopulation of rats in a box will kill each other or commit suicide. Why don't we leave off analyzing why these rats went crazy. We know they are crazy and we know that, as long as so many are in the box, they are going to keep going crazy. We can compute on top of computing and give all kinds of drugs and anything you want to put into the rats to make them survive, but sometimes it's a heck of a lot easier to change the box population.

With cities of five million people or more psychological handicaps get greater. That is where it starts. I think that the people who have been dealing with the population problem are not getting the necessary input from psychiatrists and social psychologists and I would suggest that you never go to a psychiatric convention but go to other conventions and tell your findings. You're getting better at what you do but nobody profits from it but yourselves. I still feel that we're inside the ball and we cannot project ourselves outside. Santa Barbara is a lovely community, because it is small, it's controllable. That is why I talked about the population explosion. I think that is where we have to tackle the problem. An overwhelming percentage of the mental problems that exist today in community health can probably be solved that way.

QUESTION: I'd like to ask Mr. Rozenfeld a question. As an architect, what plans do you have for the use of nontoxic substances for power? In other words, is there a place for atomic power in future plans to avoid environmental pollution?

Mr. Rozenfeld: Okay. It's a good one. We had more pollution when we had kerosene lamps in our houses than we have to-day. More people died of pollution when we did not have electricity than are dying today from smog—smog created by power plants. Let's study these facts first. People used to live thirty years, thirty-five years. I remember that statistic; just before World War II the average age in Egypt was thirty-three years of life expectancy, whereas today it is in the fifties. So let's not knock technology altogether. We have bad technology but what we need is not less technology, it's better technology. That's the first premise.

The second premise is that we all like electricity. We don't like to live in the dark and we like air-conditioning if we live in Phoenix. Well if we want electricity somebody will produce it. That is the law of the market place. The day somebody wants to shoot down the market place then I'll shoot him. We are the market place. So technology develops—develops very, very fast. The larger the metropolitan area we create, the larger the plant we need. If we did not have a city of two, three million people, we wouldn't need the big gigantic distribution and power generation systems we have and could do with pocket size systems. But we have larger populations and therefore we are talking about a symptom again and not about the cause of the disease.

Well, while we are at it, we are not going to destroy New York or Paris or Boston or Los Angeles this year. There are now several ways of getting power, but we're running out of coal, out of gas, and out of many natural resources to produce power. We cannot get rid of the smut which present power plants, with their limited pollution controls, create. We need and have new sources of energy. Nuclear plants don't pollute the air at all. They don't kill fish either. You can go down the coast of San Onofre and you'll find that fish thrive on hot water. Some species might not like it but ten other species will. One species of fish might be killed but people who need electricity will have electricity. There is a danger in nuclear energy but there is more danger crossing the street. Whatever we create, whatever kind of machine we create, there is going to be danger.

I have been involved with working on the environmental aspects of nuclear power for the last eight years. I can tell you that they are infinitely better than any other source of power we can ever have. People do not have to be afraid of this. If one blows up, and it can happen just as the mind of the person can blow up, some human beings will die. Accidents will occur, human beings will always die. Most people demand the impossible, they are instant experts who don't understand that what they are asking for might not be possible. Technology and the business community react to what the market wants in the best way they know.

MR. KELLY: What about the fusion process? Isn't it possible that if that's developed we can have power without pollution?

MR. ROZENFELD: Yes, but that will take time. That is maybe twenty to thirty-five years away. Meanwhile I don't want to live without electricity and you don't either.

DR. BIERER: I have been interested in the problem of democracy for many years. You see, democracy has only one weapon and that is to prove that it works. But does it? Speaking historically, I would like to suggest that democracy doesn't work; throughout history democracies have turned into autocracies. For that reason, I am anxious to suggest that your democracy, and even our democracy in England, might not be as strong as we think, and that our democracies might suddenly turn into autocratic systems. Now, I wonder if we can ask ourselves, "What are the fundamentals of good government?" If we can answer this question then we might be able to see what we have to provide to make our democracies work.

I hope Mr. Kelly, you will put me right, because I'm just asking questions. I thought there are three things we should try to get, that is: first, freedom; second, security; and third, motivation. These three fundamentals appear to me most important. If I look at the three leading countries; Russia, America and Great Britain, in terms of these fundamentals I would say that in your country you have a maximum of motivation. The American who is selling newspapers today believes he can be a multi-millionaire to-

morrow. I know it doesn't happen every day but theoretically
that is possible. Yet your people have a minimum of security—today a millionaire and tomorrow a pauper.

As to freedom, you don't have as much freedom as you think if
for no other reason than that you are all slaves to the Joneses.
Whenever American friends come to visit me in England, they
tell me if I drove my car in this country, I wouldn't have any patients. I always tell them that if somebody wants to consult my
car, I don't want him as a patient. Now as to Russia, I believe
that they have no freedom. They have some motivation because
of new developments and they have security—in any case more
security than you do. In Great Britain we have no motivation, we
have maximum freedom, and we have security in some areas.

Perhaps there are some other fundamentals which are more
important. In connection with this I'd like to make another observation. Having lived in a number of countries, I came to the
conclusion that psychologically speaking tradition is an important factor. Included in tradition are the mother and father
figures and their roles. It seems to me that American fathers have
relinquished their role as head of the family, and therefore I
call the American society a fatherless society. And I just wonder,
would American society be more secure if it had more tradition,
a greater role for the father in the family?

MR. KELLY: Freedom, security, and motivation. I think those
three elements are constantly changing in their relationships
and balances, particularly here. In my lifetime I've gone through
periods when we had very little motivation. During the great depression people sank into despair, there were no opportunities.
President Hoover couldn't think of anything to do and said, "Well,
it just has to go on like this, sometime it will change." This was
his doctrine. And when Mr. Roosevelt came in he appealed to a
new motivation in the American people. This in turn led to more
security, the social security system. Some people objected that the
social security system abridged our freedom. But I think we can
read these things in so many different ways. I've read many ar-
ticles about this recently, some of which attempt to demonstrate
that there is more freedom and more security in the United
States now and less motivation than we have ever had in our his-

tory. I would agree that there has been a change, for the motivation of young people today is quite different from that of people my age.

I have two sons and I have met many students through them and many students come through the Center. I really think a kind of mutation is happening in the human species. Certainly, these young people while groping around make all kinds of mistakes. Some of them go off the deep end with drugs, violence and so on. But there is something different about them that I don't find in middle-aged people. For them racism is nonsense. They have just thrown the whole racism bag overboard while many middle-aged people haven't done that. Young people talk about freedom in very different terms than we do, in terms of the freedom to be different. Kids in school don't make fun of fat kids or of those with funny faces or of those who have handicaps as they did when I went to school. There is a remarkable psychological change in these young people, and we will have to reconsider freedom, security and motivation in the light of this psychological change. Do you think there is anything to that?

DR. BIERER: Yes, there is, but we must make this change known in other countries to overcome stereotypes. Having come in contact with many communistic countries, I wondered how we can produce bridges between countries. I believe that the only bridge is direct exchange of people.

MR. KELLY: I think you can reach people when you approach each other with openness, as human beings. But if you get others defensive, if you get on political, ideological and economic questions they must defend their dogmas. To me this is one of the hopes of the world, that human beings can liberate themselves from ideologies. The young people who, I think, may move us into a totally new world are people who are largely liberated from a fixed attachment to ideology.

MR. ROZENFELD: I was intrigued with Dr. Bierer's idea about the mother and father image. Being of foreign origin and having traveled quite a bit, I am still searching for what America is. It seems to me we have a matriarchal and patriarchal society simultaneously. Some sections of the country are still patriarchal. For example, in a small town in the heart of the middle west of twen-

ty, thirty to forty people you'll find a totally patriarchal society;
but the large cities are matriarchal. There is a dichotomy in this
country. I still haven't found out what the United States is all
about. Except whenever I probe the subject, I keep coming back
to the economic structure of it and not so much to its governmental structure.

We have an economic system, free enterprise, capitalism; whether we think it good, bad, or indifferent, I don't think we have
found any better yet. One way or another we will find remedies
for our society's dilemmas only if the system is perpetuated. I
think this economic system is infinitely more important to the
solving of our social problems than the actual governmental structure.

MR. KELLY: I think you will have chaos unless you have some
political structure which can unify a huge society with 210 million people. I don't think an economic system by itself is going to
work. It will collapse.

DR. BIERER: I believe in Great Britain neither the members
of parliament nor the members of the House of Lords really look
after the nation's interest. They are looking out for their pockets,
their constituents, their parties. As I see it, in a democracy nobody looks after the interests of the whole community.

MR. KELLY: That's the same problem we have. I think our
only way to develop a community could be by a nation-wide discussion on what kind of a constitution is necessary for a nation of
continental size with 210 million people in the last third of the
twentieth century.

DR. BIERER: I just wonder if we wouldn't get further if we
could organize groups of people who are not members of an
existing political party and have no vested interests. Such a
group would be a force interested in the well-being of the total
community.

MR. KELLY: I think if television, the educational capacity of
television, could be used adequately we could develop such a
force for the well-being of the entire community. Steve Allen is
here. You have done a lot of thinking about the potentialities of
television. Do you think it could be used to bring together people
in such a way that they could care about the whole community?

Mr. Allen: The technological potential is dazzling. I think eventually you're going to have to interest men and women like the *Common Cause* people, like Ralph Nader and influential representatives of the consumer revolution in that technology. This will take the participation of many people. There is no one hero who can help nor one simple answer.

Question: Is it the system that doesn't work or is it the people that don't work? Is the ultimate responsibility on people or on the system—given the size of our land?

Mr. Kelly: There is no single answer. I would say that we don't know what people are. We're always trying to figure who we are and what we may become. Democracy or any kind of open system offers the best chance for constant experimentation, change and not being afraid of change. This is one advantage people in a democracy have over a rigid totalitarian system that we don't give up on people, we don't think people are bad. We haven't done it yet but by God we can and we will if we don't watch out.

Question: Mr. Kennedy, if an individual enters a church community, how important is it to the therapeutic value of his experience that he make a voluntary and religiously motivated commitment?

Rev. Kennedy: That's very important. The churches have reached the institutional stage where they need to have more members to keep the church running. For this reason they do not question the decision and motivation of prospective members too closely. If a person has not made a true decision about being there the following situation might occur: Some members of the congregation come along and say, "Look, we are going to change this church. What do you think?" The uncommitted congregation member might then find himself in a community he never decided to belong to. He accepted the church as a fixed place, but he made no knowledgeable and personal commitment to the community. In a changing situation he will either feel uncomfortable or he will resist change within the community and force the church to petrify. Neither solution is therapeutic for the individual and for the church. So I think it is essential that individuals clearly know the nature of their commitment so that they can feel free in the community and change with it.

PART IV
CONTEMPORARY SOCIAL PROBLEMS

Chapter 8

THE PSYCHIATRIST'S PROBLEM OF EVALUATING DEVIANT BEHAVIOR DURING RAPID SOCIAL CHANGE

NORMAN Q. BRILL, M.D.

Social Criteria

DEVIANT BEHAVIOR must be viewed from the standpoint of its meaning. Under certain circumstances, because of its meaning, it is not regarded as deviant. Killing the enemy in wartime (when it is a group sanctioned goal) is not regarded as deviant behavior. Here the refusal to kill may be considered *deviant*. Destroying the enemy is the goal of the group; it is looked upon as constructive and generally self-preservative. From a cold, objective, detached, *scientific* point of view, however, killing is killing, and circumstances do not alter facts.

In civil settings rioting, looting, disrupting, burning, shooting are usually regarded as deviant and antisocial. The persons who engage in such behavior are regarded as disturbed, disordered or delinquent, and when there is a continuing commitment to such behavior the individual is considered to be *psychopathic* and a fit subject for psychiatric examination and labeling or incarceration. It is a different matter when the rioting, looting and killing become the avowed objective of a group that is convinced that it is being mistreated and that its grievances will not be attended to or corrected unless some normally unacceptable method is employed. The illegal Boston Tea Party is viewed differently in the light of history.

Here again, the group element is crucial and, in fact, the group must be organized and large enough to maintain that its actions are not *criminal* in the way that individual rioting, looting, killing and burning would be automatically considered.

It is society then that defines normality and abnormality of behavior. It is of interest that in the final analysis insanity is still

determined by laymen rather than the professional—the psychiatrist. It can be left to judge or jury because the opinions of
one or three psychiatrists are not enough. Society decides who is
sick and who is bad. Society decides who is to be treated and who
punished.

Fighting and taunting the police, provoking violence, disrupting meetings, seizing of buildings, vandalism, detention of people
in authority, deliberately attempting to disrupt the normal functioning of a society when done for a cause are considered noble
and heroic (by the group) especially when it is known that there
is real risk of arrest or bodily damage.

The mere existence of a social goal is not enough; it has to be
successful. The Nazis and the Fascists achieved acceptance and
gratitude for their revolutionary activities from a majority of
their fellow countrymen as long as they were successful. It was only when they were defeated by others that their nefariousness was
admitted by former followers.

In addition to civil disrupters young persons who dropped or
flunked out of school, who not only did not want to work but
considered wanting to work a *hang up*, who were concerned with
the pursuit of pleasure and used drugs freely in their attempt to
achieve it and who depended on family and society for their support would have certainly been classified or diagnosed as abnormal
in the past.

However, there are increasing numbers of people who subscribe to such behavior as normal or at least defend it as *understandable*. People are being urged to *tune out*. Work for work's
sake is called abnormal. Success is something to be avoided. Pain
should be unnecessary, and being taken care of by an affluent society is being constructive by assisting in the consumption of and
not adding to the overproduction.

However, questions still arise about the nature of the behavior of political activists and the large number of students who
join and support and encourage their activities. The rebellion
against so much of the standards and mores of the establishment that is manifested in gross deviations in dress, speech, sexual
activity, attitudes toward police, honesty and styles of living sug-

gests the presence of degrees of alienation or hate that by *establishment* standards is pathological.

Increased Expectations

It is suspected by many that the *strong feeling against war* in so many students masquerades behind a facade of idealism and conscience and is little more than resentment at being interfered with, being forced to do something that doesn't fit in with their own life plans. (I have seen many who have knowingly resorted to the deception of claiming to be conscientious objectors because this was a way to get out of being drafted.) Even the expressed fear of being killed has a hollow ring when it is voiced by doctors who have a notably low mortality rate in the services, but who talk like infantrymen.

It is pointed out by some that rather than there being "increased distance on campuses between students and administration, and students and faculty," students today are a lot closer to faculty and administration and more influential than college students of 40 to 50 years ago ever dreamed of being. Authoritarianism was much more marked then than now. What has changed is the tolerance threshold. Youth is less accepting of limitations in their freedom *to do their thing,* just as much as they are less accepting of racial prejudice, poverty, hypocrisy, etc. It is a blanket or widespread attitude that applies to self interests as much as to societal interests. The generation gap involves these altered attitudes and expectations. It is the impatience, the inexplicable degree of anger, the disrespect for the old mores and standards, the intolerance, the demand for immediate gratification of whatever wish that the establishment hears loud and clear. To many the social concerns that are expressed somehow don't seem to be the sole reason.

Increased expectations appear to be associated not only with idealism but with less tolerance, more demand for immediate action or gratification and violence and demonstration as techniques for achieving action. To the traditionalist in psychiatry this behavior gives the impression of being impulse ridden or immature and thus deserving of a *name* that will characterize or classify the psychopathology.

De Tocqueville called attention to the correlation between rising expectations and social disaffection.

"The evil which was suffered patiently as inevitable seems unendurable as soon as the idea of escaping from it crosses men's minds. All the abuses then removed call attention to those that remain and they now appear more galling. The evil, it is true, has become less, but sensibility to it has become more acute."[1]

Conflicting Opinions

Donald McDonald, in an excellent article, *Youth,* points out that:

For every assertion made about American youth, there exists, it seems, an exact denial. Youth are alleged to be at once sick and sane; alienated and involved; political and apolitical; arrogant and humble; naive and sophisticated; immoral and religious; obscene and idealistic.

What strikes one observer as *youthful arrogance* seems to another *refreshing candor.* Where one critic discovers a *pathological condition* in young people, another rejoices in the sanity of youth's rejection of a *sick society.* The *anarchism* that sends shivers down the spines of some adults is welcomed by others as a sign of *healthy anti-authoritarianism.* What looks like *cultural nihilism* from one quarter, looks like the emergence of an authentic *counter-culture* from another.[2]

Bruno Bettelheim talks about rebellious youth being *fixated* at the temper tantrum stage, but Margaret Mead takes hope in "the young people who are rebelling all around the world, rebelling against whatever forms the governmental and educational systems take."[3]

Bettelheim at the Menninger Foundation in February, 1970, took the position that revolutionary behavior in young people is merely "shooting off their mouths." In the past adults regarded this as normal for their age and paid no attention to them, while waiting for them to grow up. He was appalled rather by the self-hatred of the intellectual establishment of this country and its encouraging attacks from youth while "lying down and submitting to aggression."[4]

John Spiegel is willing to consider student rebellion a realistic reaction to profound disillusionment. He believes "it is unfair and narrow to ascribe the social phenomenon of student rebellion to preexisting psychopathology and unresponsibility on the part of activist students."[5] He prefers to attribute it to Vietnam, the participation of the university in military research and training, unsatisfactory arrangements for minority-group students, the quality and pertinence of the curriculum, the limitations on student freedom and the general decision-making process. He feels it is not reasonable to raise questions about the irrational unconscious motives of students while ignoring the similar implications of the behavior of those members of the faculty and administration who oppose them. The self-esteem of many of these members is derived from their hard-won status and, therefore, is very vulnerable to the student challenge of their authority.

Spiegel's reasoning is not convincing to many who promptly point out that previous generations of students were confronted with much more realistic grounds (if present conditions are realistic causes) in the past and the frank statements of some of their leaders that their goal is radicalization of students. The issues are not important. The goal is to produce change.

Past generations had come a long way from those that preceded them and made their contributions to progress or change; parents always remarked about how different the new generation was, children seem to have never just followed in the footprints of their parents; they started leaving the farms a long time before WWII; automobiles and radio and refrigeration and telephones and electricity and modern housing and the industrial revolution were all rather startling innovations without having produced the contemporary revolt.

The conflicting opinions are highlighted by John Brooks, who in his excellent article "A Clean Break with the Past" says:

> Looked at in a favorable light, the new youth are gentle, loving, natural, intuitive, opposed only to war and obsession with money, to hypocrisy and the other agreed upon weaknesses of modern society as organized by their elders. In a different perspective they represent progressive school permissiveness and self-indulgence run wild. Their causes are merely self-serving (opposition to the draft, for example). Their attitudes are self-righteous ("just because you are growing older do not be afraid of change," they gravely lecture their parents and teachers). Their manners are deplorable or non-

existent. Their minds are flabby, their herding together indicates fear of standing alone, and the manner of their protests sometimes appears ominously anti-democratic.[6]

Giving a stranger a flower or a jelly bean somehow doesn't convey the feeling of love that it is supposed to; rather it seems naivè, childlike and often play-acting.

The childlike qualities of seeing things as black or white, impatience, demands, and symbolic gifts, seems to be consistent with the trend to regress to the more primitive in dress, speech, music and living, away from the more complicated civilized and controlled life.

Some would have us believe that the intensity of reaction against racism is related to and a function of the amount of racism. Others insist there is a lot less racism today than there was fifty years ago. What there is, isn't tolerated as much. The same can be said about poverty.

It's easier to see the hypocrisy in society (in others) than in oneself, and hidden beneath the intolerance of society's realistic shortcomings are comparable ones in the youths who are most articulate in their condemnations.

The mechanisms of denial, projection and regression are clear cut—whether a name is put on them or not.

They want fun. They want to do work that they enjoy but have problems finding. They don't want to work as a means to an end, to plow a field in order to get corn next year. They want to enjoy the plowing, the harvesting and the shucking.

Suggested Explanations

Many have attributed this complex change to increased permissiveness, greater honesty, affluence, population increase, technological development, the threat of an atomic holocaust, increased communications and speed and ease of travel.

Ardrey sees overcrowding, reduction in personal space, enlarging human organizations, loss of self identity, inadequate philosophy, animal xenophobia, boredom of increased economic security and a need for stimulation as basic factors in today's violence.[7]

Overlooked, perhaps, is the fact that for many years now we

have witnessed increasing emphasis on individuality and self-expression that was coincident with pressures for greater conformity which increased density of population demanded—a combination that could hardly result in anything but confusion or schizophrenia.

Our improved and altered socioeconomic situation changed the sense of importance children experienced with their parents. Children were no longer needed for their help; at the same time, they became greater burdens to their parents who catered to them in ways never before seen. The children were made to feel important and unimportant at the same time.

Industrialization and division of labor gave little feeling of pride to those who could never experience the satisfaction of creativity. Occupational groups competed with each other for greater portions of the country's annual production.

Increasingly, less and less people knew or had any contact with their governmental representatives who played such important roles in determining what their lives would be like. More and more individuals experienced a feeling of decreasing control over their futures after having been led to believe they could control the world as they had their parents.

They were bombarded by dramatized reports of the unusual day and night by the newspapers, TV and radio and could not help but develop concern that everything was going to pot or getting ready to explode.

In addition there is the increased period of dependence with more years of education, the advent of the peace-time draft, sanctioning and encouragement of credit financing (even for education) and with a shorter work week—talk of the need to prepare oneself for leisure time activities.

Altered attitudes toward work are seen by some as a consequence of a change in the nature and meaning of work. According to Morgan:

"new technocracy has made the whole idea of working for a living obsolete. The nature of work has already been changed by automation. At least two or three times during his lifetime technocracy is likely to overtake him and render his skills at work irrelevant and wasteful. Many activities as in the expanded service industries that would not have been called work by our grandfathers are now regarded as highly legitimate. Demand is more and more for a guaranteed income. Attitudes toward work will have to change."[8]

Hoke believes that in America at least, the individual's goal is no longer to fend off hunger, but to stave off meaninglessness in all life's facets including both work and leisure. "When work is no longer a self-fulfilling activity, anxiety arises and men flee from work to leisure and compulsive consumption."[9]

There are those like John Brooks who see the altered behavior of youth as an understandable (and natural?) outgrowth of the explosive transformation in the technical and political aspects of life. Brooks believes that the present altered American mood has had no precedents or antecedents; it represents to him almost a clear break; it seems to have come out of the blue.

Only the younger half of the American people (under 28) have never known the world of traditional values as it was without the disrupters of those values—television, computers, jet travel, space travel and the threat of nuclear extinction. Only the younger half truly belong to the new world because they have not any old world to compare it with.

So it comes about that the elders, whether they conservatively wring their hands over the new changes or liberally try to understand, absorb and temper them, feel like expatriate visitors in their own country . . . those born in the years immediately after V-J Day who were entering college when the Vietnam War was escalated, are leaving it now, and who have lived only in the strange new world can scarcely be expected to go back where they have never been.[10]

He is convinced that the end of the war will not bring with it a returning to the familiar and an end to problems, but a pushing forward to something new and unknown.

The Psychiatrist's Dilemma

The increased pressure and insistence on individuality and nonconformity as a sign of health has created confusion in the traditional, establishment-oriented person who was brought up to believe that the individual who behaved and dressed in a bizarre way and took no pride in his appearance or accomplishments had something wrong with him.

It is interesting to see how young people have been quick to denounce the placing of diagnostic labels on nonconformists, while at the same time they have been responsible for the belittling, name calling and labelling of conservatives and law enforcing people (squares, pigs, etc.).

The young person who doesn't *conform* to the dress and spirit of the rebellious is now self-conscious and defensive. If a college boy doesn't try *pot* the others want to know what's the matter with him. Sexual restraint, too, is increasingly regarded as *pathological*.

It has been said that there is no conformity that exceeds that of the so-called nonconformist, that it is difficult to tell them apart with their faces so uniformly hidden behind beards, their feet bare or protruding from sandals or booted, their hair long, their clothes unpatterned, riding their motorcycles or buses or carrying a guitar.

This is not to imply that all who appear this way *are* the same —in fact there is an insistence that each one be recognized as an individual, different from others and worthwhile for himself rather than for his conformity or appearance. To them it's in the service of avoiding the *anonymity* of the gray suit and cleanly shaved face.

As compared with other physicians, psychiatrists tend to be anti-authoritarian, politically liberal and more actively concerned with social problems and issues. They are more apt than others to call society *sick* and to be divided in attributing emotional illness to deficiencies in the person himself and to external societal stresses.

So far psychiatrists have not been called upon, at least in civilian settings, to diagnose or label these behaviors. If labels were to be given they would vary with the personal standards and political beliefs of the psychiatrists. The diagnosis of heart disease or cancer does not change with the times or the personal biases of the physicians. This is not the case with psychiatric disorders and psychiatrists. We are appalled to learn that political deviants in certain communist countries are regarded as mentally ill. We are not as appalled with the widely held notions that there is something seriously wrong with the leaders and followers of the radical and revolutionary movements who have been creating so much commotion in the United States. Opinions are divided whether these *troublemakers* should be in jail, under the care of psychiatrists, or hailed and encouraged as the saviors of our society.[11]

Dr. Seymour Halleck, Professor of Psychiatry at the University of Wisconsin, asked how you can classify restless students when 12,000 of them march in an illegal parade to protest the absence of a black studies program.

He feels that even if the war in Vietnam ended tomorrow the unrest would continue. He believes the anger over the draft and the efforts to avoid it have carried a lot of shame and guilt so that after four years the student not only begins to despise the war, but the university that has protected him from it, along with the country that has created the situation and often himself; all of which probably contributes to overt, angry, and often illegal student protest.

But, he continues: When the rate of change becomes too fast, people simply despair of trying to adapt to it. They simply despair of trying to plan for the future. They just begin to live in the present and do it now. "If you're sailing on the S.S. *Titanic* you might as well go First Class." The inability to plan for the future used to be one of the hallmarks of the *psychopath*.

Halleck found that many of the youths who come to the psychiatrist are charming at first, but about the third or fourth hour they have nothing to say. They have lost all depth and are actually empty.[12]

Robert E. Gould considers the questions, is youth *troubled* or *in trouble?* Are they rebellious, deviant and disturbed, or are they concerned about and alarmed by evils of society?

He believes that the life style of the hippie with his love ethic is expressed in his exhortation *do your thing,* which means do whatever is right for you so long as it fulfills your potential needs and does not interfere with another person fulfilling his potential needs. "This leads to the anti-intellectual stance of so many hippies who believe that over-mechanization and decreased personalization of life have obscured man's ability to be in touch with his own real feelings. He uses drugs, music and meditation to find himself and a meaning to his life."[13]

Gould believes that the *dropping out* of society of the hippie is active rather than passive behavior. While it might be evidence of a high level of anxiety, it reflects courage and strength in its going against the mainstream with its irrelevant values and mores. He regards their *dropping out* not only a flight from an environment that is felt to be oppressive but confrontation and defiance meant to change it. He adds that while many hippies may be individually sick, their movement as a whole is socially healthy.

A different opinion is expressed by Voge who, while recognizing the rebellious aspect of the drug culture, reminds us that the ultimate sanction against the rebellious youth in the past was economic. If the parents refused to support him he had no choice except to starve or to go to work. But today dropouts can survive without their parents' support. He quotes Romeo who has worked with many youngsters and who says "kids have discovered they can live on the offal of society. They don't have to *make something of themselves.* Food, clothing and shelter are no longer matters to worry about. Kids can live on welfare, or go to the Salvation Army or a free store for help."[14]

Voge believes that the Vietnam war, alienation and a so-called plastic unhuman society may incline youngsters toward trying drugs, but the trigger is a very personal one. He sees some using drugs to maintain social contact, others to withdraw, and others to see *how far they can go* with no normal concern for their existence.

The psychiatrist's job is to assist people who are having problems of adjusting and functioning because of emotional problems. In his attempts to help persons face and deal with reality, he is regarded by many as an agent of the establishment who tries to assist patients to adjust to the culture.[15]

This presumes that he (the psychiatrist) is identified with the culture. The conservative American psychiatrist would look upon rebellion of young people in the Soviet Union as normal, understandable and something to be encouraged. In this he reveals his own politico-social philosophy which exists even though he is unaware of it in his dealing with patients, and he generally is more liberal than his medical colleagues.

He was reared in a culture that placed a high value on individual enterprise, hard work, competition and financial, social and occupational success. He was not indoctrinated, as are the young in communist countries, to have a concern for the common good, to think of what is best for society, and to feel that his primary obligation is to others and not to himself. What religious attitudes he learned from parents, ministers, or absorbed from the culture, taught him to be concerned for others, to love his fellow man, to be his brother's keeper, to be charitable, help the weak, the sick and the poor, but this is somewhat different from the doctrine of socialism.

His approach to patients, despite efforts to maintain a detached neutrality, was bound to reflect his biases and his education. His theoretical constructs were bound to be different from the Soviet psychiatrist to whom societal responsibility was the *sine qua non* and who would see as his goal of treatment restoration of the individual to a productive state in which he could made his contribution and fulfill his obligation to society.

This just exemplifies the lack of specificity in psychopathology. What is abnormal or pathological in one culture or time is not necessarily so in another culture or another time where there might be great differences in ways of dealing with basic instinctual impulses, mores and customs, and feelings of self-importance.

The social obligations of scientists and their research have in recent times become a subject of increasing concern as a consequence of the aftermath of the atomic bomb. Today there is concern about the implications of the isolation of a pure gene. It is not left to the scientists to consider whether their discoveries will in the long run lead to more evil than good or to decide how their findings will be used.

During times of rapid socio-cultural change when mores and political philosophies are being modified, it becomes very difficult to apply the same *traditional* criteria of psychopathology. Reality itself is changing. Farnsworth states that "some of the young have become so critical that they have moved beyond the usual forms of protest and have become alienated from society and lost much of their commitment to academic values and intellectual achievement."[16] He quotes Keniston that psychologic disturbances are common among them. He partly blames the permissive mode of childrearing in the U.S. for the demand for immediate gratification of desires and goals. He maintains that in addition they were taught to be both idealistic and critical but "not taught to balance *all* the rights and values involved in a particular situation."[17] The glaring discrepancy between the ideals they were taught and the ethical practices they observed in *respectable persons* became apparent, but their lack of discipline and unwillingness or inability to sustain action mean that when they encounter opposition they have no constructive techniques for dealing with it and they react with fear, anger and violence.

Yet he maintains that labelling today's activist college students mentally ill "is not justified and in fact it might be argued convincingly that the nature of this dissatisfaction connotes a higher than usual level of mental health in the realm of concern for others."[18] He has also commented on the difficulties of the college psychiatrist in this period of campus unrest when revolutionary forces have begun to advocate destruction of the universities.[19]

He maintains that the radicals are not *necessarily sick*. Their strong feelings about difficult problems often motivate inappropriate behavior. He believes the psychiatrist can best assist them in channeling their idealism into appropriate action, rather than pass judgment on ideals or goals. He should devote himself to helping the various factions understand one another better and to helping those students who are engaging in self-defeating behavior. He warns that trying to achieve rapport with patients by over-identifying with them is a mockery of effective physician-patient rapport.

The problem is: What is *inappropriate behavior?* What was appropriate behavior at the time of the American Revolution, the French Revolution or the Communist Revolution? Ignoring for the moment whether it is right or wrong for the psychiatrist to stay uninvolved, one can ask, "is it possible for the psychiatrist to remain aloof from a world that is changing all around him?" It was not too long ago that some psychiatrists had to flee from Nazi Germany, not because they were Jews, but because their practices had become inimical to the State. How can one claim freedom of approach in treating psychiatric patients in Red China or the Soviet Union?

Rubenstein describing the community mental health centers during civil disorders relates how they sometimes were used as shelters or for emergency food distribution, i.e. for disaster relief and sometimes for the convenience of the police as a staging area or as a holding area for violators. He reported that "even the most neutral and dispassionate nonrelated activities may leave a center vulnerable to criticism. For instance, a center which had engaged in seemingly noncontroversial relief work during the riot, usually in close collaboration with municipal authorities, viewed as quite ominous a memo sent to them several weeks later by the state agency of which they are a part, reminding them of a federal statute which threatens to withhold federal funds from a recipient providing 'services or assistance' to anyone convicted of 'carrying on' a riot."[20]

Szasz warns us against considering difference from the norm or majority as deviant (this includes mental patients) when deviance implies sick and mental illness. He reminds us how Benjamin Rush, the father of American Psychiatry, regarded as a form of insanity (Anarchia) "the excess of passion for liberty, inflamed by the successful issue of the war (after the peace of 1783) that produced in many people opinions and conduct which could not be removed by reason nor restrained by government."[21] Szasz somewhat contemptuously views Rush as considering the protection of property and morals as a medical problem and preservation of the puritan ethic as a medical concern.[22] He stresses the tendency to transform social problems into medical problems in modern totalitarian states (both national socialist and communist) in order to identify, stigmatize and control particular segments of the population. He is concerned about the possibility of the psychiatrist emerging as a political evangelist, social activist and medical despot whose role is to protect the state from the troublesome citizen.[23] He recalls that psychiatrists in Nazi Germany played a leading role in developing gas chambers whose first victims were mental patients.

So far there has been little tendency to *diagnose* alienated youth. In fact, violence, disruption and dropping out have had considerable support and acceptance. The mental health drop-out rates and suicide rates of college students have changed very little over the past four decades.[24]

Several major institutions reported a marked falling off in psychiatric case loads during demonstrations.[25]

Yet, psychiatrists are repeatedly asked "what is the matter with the young people today?" It is not difficult to conceive of dedicated disturbers of the peace who commit acts of violence being regarded as maladjusted and as fit subjects for the psychiatrist. While I don't subscribe to Szasz's total rejection of involuntary hospitalization, I believe he has some cause for concern that moral and political issues will be dealt with as medical or psychiatric.

If we are going to have a planned economy and if the good of the individual is to be equated with (and subservient to) the good of the State (and there is evidence that we are moving rapidly in that direction), dissent and particularly aggressive or violent dissent may indeed be viewed as deviant and, therefore, in need of treatment if not punishment.

However, we are also confronted with the ill effects of the competitiveness of our society, overpopulation, pollution, nationalism, technology and overproduction, the vulnerability of the megapolis as a consequence of its dependence on so many factors outside of itself for its functioning and survival, poverty, racism and immoral wars; the possibility of man destroying himself with the A Bomb, and feelings of impotence along with the frustration that accompanies it when government or the establishment at any level remains unresponsive to these concerns are real.

What then should the position of the psychiatrist be? He should realize that although there are psychodynamic underpinnings to the behavior of the activist, rebellious youth, this is not reason to assume they are sick and to give them *psychiatric names*. There are, of course, borderline or psychotic or paranoid individuals who attach themselves to any movement. They are recognized as such by their associates and utilized as long as they are effective. But for the most part, the activist is distributed along a continuum from the idealist to the fanatic. Some are

more politically motivated than others. Some are even more respectful than others. In short, there is not one personality that is
characteristic of the activist.

With the concern about overpopulation, pollution, the exhaus-
tion of natural resources, and the altered attitudes about sex,
families, patriotism and work, it is difficult to describe behavior
of the young anti-establishment activist as immature, because
he doesn't work, isn't interested in getting married and having a
family. He regards his *not going along with current mores* as being
motivated by socially constructive principles rather than selfish-
ness, or laziness as he is apt to be regarded.

The psychiatrist should be aware of the dangers of generalizing
about the meaning and significance of any behavioral phenomenon, especially in time of active social change. He should be
mindful that there are many examples of political leaders who
had obvious psychopathology and that their personality disturbances didn't seem to interfere with their popularity and success.

Psychiatrists seem all too eager to place *labels* on political figures
as they did in the famous Goldwater questionnaire. They turned
out to look pretty silly.

Regardless of motivation, society will hold people responsible
for their antisocial or criminal activity however sincere the motives may have been. Kidnapping, bombing, or other use of force
will not be tolerated by governmental agencies charged with enforcing the law and maintaining the peace.[26] It may be of interest that in communist countries, inability to adjust to the social structure is considered the main cause of mental illness.

It may be that some activists, radicals, revolutionists, traitors,
or dropouts will be referred for psychiatric examination by the
courts (as in the case of Ezra Pound) or at the insistence of their
families because of behavior that is regarded as deviant.

Some may be found ill. By current standards they may have
personalities that could be considered disordered and immature,
antisocial, paranoid, obsessed, amoral or schizoid. They might be
characterized as impulse ridden, impatient or fanatical. They
might have one of the many varieties of psychoneurotic disorders
or even be psychotic. It is essential that each person be indi-

vidually examined and evaluated. Uncooperativeness and even contempt for psychiatrists does not automatically indicate psychopathology. Oscar Lewis demonstrated very dramatically how different members of a family perceived and explained an identical incident differently. Psychiatrists may be perceived differently by persons of varying convictions.

The psychiatrist must avoid being influenced by his own biases. When he examines someone who has committed a crime that may have been associated with strong political convictions and been part of some activist group effort to effect some social change, he can do no more than report his findings. It is not for the psychiatrist to determine the person's responsibility. It is his job to describe the person's mental status: the nature and degree of any disorder in thinking or intelligence, in impulse control, in affect and mood and the developmental chain of events that are relevant. Organic as well as psychological factors should be explored. He can give his estimate of the extent to which the person knew what he was doing, planned what he did, and was able to resist his impulses. The psychiatrist functions as a medical expert, not as a judge, jury or prosecutor.

If psychopathology is found it will still not automatically indicate whether a person's actions were symptomatic of his emotional disorder and as a consequence (if one were to follow the implications of the Durham Decision) not truly something for which they could be held legally responsible.

Much as one would like to deal with social unrest, or revolution as one would deal with a disturbed person it just hasn't been possible. These must be considered from a different perspective that involves the application of principles of social psychiatry. In the armed forces, the rate of psychiatric breakdowns was found to be related to the quality of leadership, *esprit de corps,* fair rewards and punishment, adequacy of training, expectancy of relief from excessive stress, and a host of other variables in the life of the soldier. The psychiatrist in civilian settings is obliged to recognize those elements that are causing emotional disturbances and to attempt to get society to correct them. His greatest contribution can be to determine whether in fact poverty, inadequate diets, housing, racism are producing disturbances in individuals, whether lack of identity, alienation, affluence, technological developments, pollution, war, etc. are the basis of poor morale and then do all he can to call society's attention to the factors along with suggested solutions.

As Ardrey has advised "the survival of the violent subgroups is threatened by their dependence on the existing social structure and a biological need for order." He sees the need for compromise, providing prizes of identity, negotiation and correction of genuine injustices. Otherwise he predicts that someone else will rule the men who cannot agree on how to rule themselves.[27]

BIBLIOGRAPHY

1. Quoted by Richardson, Secretary of H.E.W.: In *Drug Research Report*, 13(29):S-2, July 22, 1970.
2. McDonald, D.: Youth. *The Center Magazine*, 3:22-33, 1970.
3. McDonald: *Op. cit.*
4. *Menninger Perspective:* 1(2):23-25, 1970.
5. Spiegel, J.: Frontiers of Hospital Psychiatry. Nutley, New Jersey, Roche Laboratories, 7, #3, 1970.
6. Brooks, J.: A Clean Break with the Past. *American Heritage*, 21:72, 1970.
7. Ardrey, R.: The Violent Way. *Life Magazine*, 69:56c, 1970.
8. Morgan, J. S.: Work or Non-Work. *Archives of Environmental Health*, 17:3-5, 1968.
9. Hoke, B.: The Meaning of Work: Contemporary Views Reviewed. *Archives of Environmental Health*, 16:598-603, 1968.
10. Brooks, J.: *op. cit.*, pp. 22-23.
11. There are differences of opinion even among Africans about whether the Black Panthers are criminals or freedom fighters. Meisler, S.: *Los Angeles Times*, Section A, p. 19, January 3, 1971.
12. Halleck, Seymour, M.D.: Personal Communication.
13. Gould, R. E.: Troubled Youth in Psychiatry. *Medical World News*, p. 56, 1969.
14. Voge, A. J.: Why Youngsters Join the High Society. *Hospital Physician*, p. 35, August, 1970.
15. T. Szasz, in a speech at the Twentieth Anniversary Celebration of Dianetics and Scientology in Long Beach, California, July, 1970, demanded a war on Institutional Psychiatry, maintaining that it was one of the most important enemies of individual dignity and freedom.
16. Farnsworth, D. L.: *Mental Health Scope*, 4(20):8, 1970.
17. Farnsworth: Mental, *op. cit.*

18. Farnsworth, D. L.: Annual Discourse—Youth in Protest. *New England Journal of Medicine*, 282:1235, 1970.
19. Farnsworth, D. L.: University Psychiatrist Looks at Campus Protest. *Psychiatric Opinion*, 6:6-11, 1969.
20. Rubenstein, Marc A.: *Mental Health Scope*, 4(13):3-5, 1970.
21. Szasz, T.: *The Manufacture of Madness*. New York, Harper and Row, 1970, p. 144.
22. Szasz: *op. cit.*, p. 144.
23. Szasz: *op. cit.*, p. 214.
24. Farnsworth, D. L.: Annual, *op. cit.*
25. Student Services Annual Report, UCLA, p. 36, 1969-70.
26. According to the President's Commission on Campus Unrest, "the right to dissent is not the right to resort to violence," and S. B. Robitscher insists "that the constitutional right of individuals to hold their own opinions and to act according to their own dictates must have some limit." *Medical Opinion and Review*, 5:9, 1969.
27. Ardrey, R.: *op. cit.*

Chapter 9

BLACK PEOPLE IN A
WHITE MAN'S CULTURE

PRICE M. COBBS, M.D.

MY TOPIC WAS *Black People in a White Man's Culture,* but since many of us go to conferences and hear papers all day long, I thought I would try to relate this topic more personally to you here and relate it to the conference theme *Collaboration for Mental Health.* At the San Francisco Medical Center for about three years, we have been doing a series of groups that we call *Racial Confrontation Groups.* These groups are run according to techniques adapted from traditional group psychotherapy and from various educational seminar methods, while integrating some of the newer concepts of encounter groups.

One of the things that we learned very quickly in our groups was how ignorant, how truly ignorant, people are of each other.[1] And I should say I realized with surprise (although it really would not be true surprise), all too often the professionals, the teachers, psychiatrists, psychologists, social workers, and rehabilitation therapists, were the most ignorant of other people. Many times we heard blacks described and talked glibly about by whites who knew nothing about them. Many times we heard people describe Chicano-Mexican Americans and some of their problems when these people had no knowledge of the Chicano experience. This made me think what specific measures we could take to get professionals—all of us who are sworn to serve other people—to make that necessary, serious, and scholarly effort to find out about experiences which differ from our own.

I'll never forget how shocked I was, a few days after the assassination of Dr. King, when I listened to a supposedly erudite position of a fellow worker at the San Francisco Medical Center who gave an analysis of the event based on misinformation, lack of facts, and distortion. Yet as a professional he could speak with an authority that belied his lack of knowledge.

As we talked about it, this incident made me and those around me devote ourselves to becoming more knowledgeable, more scholarly about the people with whom and for whom we work. We decided that if we were going to work with Chicano groups we would have an obligation to learn Spanish, that if we were going to work with a black group, we would not assume that because we were black, we knew all about that experience, but we would need, as part of our scholarly discipline, to learn more about it. And this is something that I certainly exhort all of you to do. As you look through the audience and see the absence of those who are different from you—that you include this resolve into the meaning of the workshop, and into the meaning of collaboration for mental health.

The profession of mental health, in looking at it broadly, at this time is bursting with new advances, new ideas, new techniques; and yet, from my vantage point, most of the old problems remain. Sometimes around the medical school I can see new machines, new drugs, and new fabrics and hear that we are on the threshold of so many new discoveries; and yet again the same nagging kind of problems remain in this country. Poverty is still the number one killer in the United States. Practically every disease that you are discussing here, every character disorder, every learning problem, is related to and has a greater incidence, greater morbidity among the poor than among the more affluent. Everything from childbirth to death is influenced adversely by being poor in an affluent country. We could go on; any of the diseases, heart disease, hypertension, schizophrenia, all affect the poor in larger numbers; and we certainly should add mental illness to this list.

Rather than avoiding the point, I wish to stress that underlying all of this is racism. And I think by any definition, racism remains the number one health problem facing this country today. I think this is something we need to ponder as we talk about black people in a white culture. Several years ago when I was serving as a consultant to the Joint Commission of Mental Health of Children in Washington, D.C., we had consultants from a variety of groups. We had consultants who were Indian and who had taught Indian children on reservations; we had several Chicanos who had worked in the project in Albuquerque, New Mexico; we had several black consultants. We were to come up with some of the major problems in the mental health of the children whom we were seeing and to whom we related.

As we came up with first one list of causes and then another, we could not escape the conclusion that racism, rather than being a term, rather than being a label, racism consisting of the inherent ideas, attitudes, feelings of most white Americans to those who are non-white, was the number one health problem which faced the children with whom we dealt.

As we become more aware of the dimensions and implications of this number-one health problem, it behooves people like you to begin to think about its relation to—not especially to what you're doing here at the conference—but about its relation to you on Monday morning when you go back to work in your regular job.

I have long since divested myself of the notion that people who come to conferences fully realize the problem I am concerned with. I'll put it another way. This morning as the young teacher mentioned innovations she would like to see in education, she assumed that people at this workshop knew what educational problems in need of innovation she meant. I can't make that assumption. All too often people at conferences don't know my problems. All too often as we talk of those major social problems which create inter-psychic problems, those major problems which we see crippling our patients, our friends, our families, we realize that the people at conferences such as this don't know about them. The people here are not doing things about them. So again, as we relate to collaboration in mental health, I would ask you to ponder my charge.

One of the things I am convinced of is that if we do not—people such as you in this room, including those of us who profess to love this country and its institutions so much—if we do not find alternatives in our culture to racism, we are going to see our country and our people destroy itself. And it is on these alternatives that, as mental health professionals, as teachers, as concerned people, I would like you to focus in the noon workshops, and more importantly, back in your work on Monday morning.

I can think of no more positive way to talk about collaboration for mental health, no choice more consistent with the commitment to help people, than to state clearly your position on some of the immoralities of our world. These are things like Vietnam, like poverty, like racism, things that go on in your various institutions and organizations which all too often you decry and yet are never quite willing to take an open stand on. I consider this, in 1971, as part of the job of a professional, namely to take a stand on issues which affect the people with whom you deal.

As professionals in thinking about collaboration, you might begin by honestly confronting yourselves, your thoughts, your attitudes, your behavior toward those human beings whom you profess to help but with whom you do not live, with whom your children do not go to school. What are your thoughts, your behavior in terms of beginning to reduce racism in this country? If you honestly confront yourself and if you are a professional, sworn and committed to help, then you have to take a vow that you will not be neutral. Once you begin to understand the causes of your students' and your patients' difficulties, once you are concerned about the welfare of your clients, you cannot be neutral.

I would think in 1971 people like you must all become advocates if you are to collaborate. I would think in 1971 people such as you must speak rather than be silent. I would think that people such as you must agitate and counsel on behalf of those who are powerless, those who are not represented here. You must do this because the changes the powerless ask for and have asked for for decades affect their mental health. I would like to think of new advocates, new kinds of collaborators. The kind of collaborators who know that more than black people have been niggerized in this country. I think we have niggerized mental patients as we were talking about them this morning, degrading them, segregating them off in hospitals and locking them up. We have niggerized people in many teaching institutions, where human beings are seen as interesting cases, teaching material. And we know that when students see human beings, including themselves, in this way, they are taught the subordination that sets up superiority and inferiority.

I think we have a very urgent job to do because our culture has now embarked on what has historically been fatal for any culture, namely to war on its young. Anyone who reads history knows that it is impossible for a culture to survive when that culture begins to war on its young. This is a burgeoning movement that we can observe and hear talked about by people from the vice-president on down. I would think that if in your communities the police brutalize black and brown people, then the advocate, the new collaborator, knows that this brutalization bears some relationship to the mental health and mental illness of these people. And the new collaborator is as much against this and says so as he or she is against any other form of illness. I would think the new collaborator, I am assuming that you who come to a workshop of this type want to be collaborators, is a healer and is not afraid to say so. The new collaborator in this culture to me is not a technician, but a person who shares his compassion as well as his skill. So I ask you to ponder what you mean by collaboration for mental health. Are you willing to look for those pockets of pathology around you, are you willing to seek them out and to begin to change?

I think once you do this, in addition to whatever oath you have taken in your professions, you must also share the oath of oppressed people. And that is, that you must commit yourself to remove oppression wherever and however you find it. Sometimes this takes more courage than some of us can muster, but if we are going to begin to talk to each other, to take note, to pick up new information, and to use it when we go back Monday morning, then we must really take this oath now.

I was listening to the radio this morning in the hotel and heard a broadcast which said that sixty percent of the people in the country who are white and mostly middle class are now supposed to be fed up with black and brown and poor and young protest. And another thing the newscaster added was that these middle class people are the first to talk about love of country, law and order, decency and morality. I would encourage you to go out among these people, to risk their censure, and to talk about what you heard here over these three days, about collaboration for mental health, for this is where a collaboration is sorely needed. I will close and give you the last lines of our book *Black Rage*, which I think were and are prophetic, which were and are very germane to the kind of world in which we live and the alternatives for that world if we do not find solutions.

> For there are no more psychological tricks blacks can play upon themselves to make it possible to exist in dreadful circumstances. No more lies can they tell themselves. No more dreams to fix on. No more opiates to dull the pain. No more patience. No more thought. No more reason. Only a welling tide risen out of all those terrible years of grief, now a tidal wave of fury and rage, and all black, black as night.[2]

BIBLIOGRAPHY

1. Editor's italics.
2. Grier, William H., and Cobbs, Price M.: *Black Rage*. New York, Basic Books, Inc., 1968, p. 213.

Chapter 10

TOWARD A NEW PHASE IN CORRECTIONAL MANAGEMENT

BURTON KERISH

Introduction

NEW RESEARCH needs have been introduced into the present phase of correctional management. This paper deals with a first attempt to study an innovative treatment approach with acting-out delinquents. The method utilized was demonstration with some attempt at objective behavior measurement. Demonstration was seen as the first really practical research method by prison administrators because it satisfied a need for active inmate involvement during incarceration while attempting to explore practical solutions to correctional treatment problems.

The inapplicability of many studies in corrections stems from highly theoretical orientation. Such projects confirm or deny hypotheses which may have little direct implications for programs, while it is program oriented research which holds the most interest for the practicing correctional worker.

The impetus for the following study came from a practical severe problem confronting the staff at the Old National Training School for Boys. The problem involved a hard core group, difficult to manage youths who obviously were not reached positively by the institutional program. A new approach for coping with these offenders was needed as they were not benefiting from rehabilitative efforts being made and their disruptive behavior drew a disproportionate amount of staff time from the rest of the population. Correctional personnel were placed in the position of spending less time with the more amenable inmates in order to cope with the intractable ones.

The program for effectively reaching these acting out delinquent youths was developed in collaboration with Dr. Herbert C. Quay, Professor of Clinical Psychology, then at the University of Illinois. Dr. Quay had been conducting research at the National Training School directed at identifying dimensions of delinquency. Utilizing the research instruments he developed, it became possible to identify difficult to manage youths early in their institutional stay. Dr. Quay's theories also tied in with other research which suggested the needs of these problem youths, and the types of programs which might meet these needs.

There is a great deal of concern in corrections about providing treatment programs for different types of delinquents. In sharp contrast, however, there is a noticeable lack of study attention given to resolving three important problems. One problem is the absence of a practical instrument which would provide a valid and reliable classification of delinquent subtypes and which could be easily administered. The second involves the tendency to eliminate from consideration a group of hardcore recidivists, who, because of acting out behavior and/or violent past histories, cannot be used. Removing this group is undoubtedly expedient but this avoids confrontation with a significant offender group.

The third problem also arises when hardcore individuals are excluded from correctional programs. This prevents a full trial being given to treatment approaches which might succeed with this type of offender. Developing effective approaches for these difficult to manage youths is a necessity. Project R.E.A.D.Y. (Reaching Effectively Acting-Out Delinquent Youths) was a first attempt to devise a program to meet this need.

Prior to the beginning of Project R.E.A.D.Y. on July 5, 1967, all youths 15 to 18 committed to the National Training School for Boys participated in the same general type of treatment program. It consisted basically of a half-day of academic school, a half-day of vocational training and participation in a counseling program during the evenings and on weekends. The counseling program was conducted by full-time correctional officer counselors under close professional supervision.

It is evident that offenders differ in their responses to the institutional regimen. Some respond well, some indifferently and others actively resist attempts to rehabilitate them. If the correctional workers could determine to which group an individual belonged shortly after his admission, more specific treatment and management programs could be planned to meet differential needs. For several years, Dr. Quay did a continuing research project at NTS. Having developed a method for differentiating delinquent persons (based on information obtained the first two weeks of confinement) he attempted to predict later institutional and post institutional behavior. The base for the research was provided by a theoretical statement by Quay relating extreme acting out (psychopathic) behavior to the need for seeking more varied sensory inputs than the environment usually provides.[1]

The nature of this pathological stimulation seeking also was investigated in experimental studies in which the more psychopathic delinquents were shown to be more susceptible to the effects of boredom, to prefer complexity to simplicity in usual form, and to chose the incongruous over the more everyday type of situation.[2] Thus a program which would provide change, varied activities, and would avoid unfilled time intervals leading to boredom was hypothesized to reduce the necessity for the psychopathic individual to create his own excitement through acting out behavior.[3]

Three questionnaires were developed to obtain information from different points of view on each newly admitted individual: one rating, made by the boy's counselor, was based on observed present behavior; a second rating based on past case history information was made by the caseworker;[4] and the third information was a test taken by the boy himself.[5] Based on material these three instruments provided there are several ways that boys can be categorized.

The method employed in this study assigns individuals in terms of the relationship between two dimensions that are present in all three questionnaires, psychopathy (P) and neuroticism (N). Using standard scores a number of times P exceeds N classifies boys into one of four groups: If P is greater than N on all three instruments, the individual is in group 3; if P exceeds N for any two ratings, that individual is in group 2; if P is higher than N for any one rating, the individual is in group 1; if P is not greater than N on any instrument, that individual is in group Zero. Thus the higher the group number 0 to 3, the more *psychopathic* the individual.

Prior research demonstrated the poor adjustment of high P individuals (groups 2 and 3).[6] For example, high P offenders have a higher rate of AWOLs and disciplinary transfers: 52 percent for groups 2 and 3, 17 percent for groups Zero and 1; they have a lower rate of parole: 24 percent for groups 2 and 3 compared with 71 percent paroled for groups Zero and 1. The high P groups have a greater number of commitments to the segregation unit: 94 percent for groups 2 and 3 as opposed to 71 percent for groups Zero and 1; and this group averages three times as many days in segregation: a mean of 40.4 days for groups 2 and 3 compared with a mean of 15.5 days for groups Zero and 1.

These, and similar data, make it clear that the high P group was not responding positively to the current institutional program. Although some problems are also evident with other groups, the high P individuals had the least success. Thus, concern was focused on this group and Project R.E.A.D.Y. was established. Its initial goal was to find a method for effectively managing high P youths so they might benefit more from institutional correctional programs; e.g., academic education and vocational training. In the NTS program, the individuals managed to evade treatment efforts by removing themselves from these rehabilitation programs. They accomplished this by frequent and lengthy segregation commitments and ultimately removed themselves from the institution by disciplinary transfer or going AWOL. The assumption was made that the institution had something worthwhile to offer these youths if they could be kept active as participants in the variety of available programs. The goal was to develop methods for effective management of the high Ps and thereby give these therapeutic programs a better chance to succeed.

Initial Phase

The program operated seven days a week and because of this, the type of youths involved, and the number and variety of activities planned, the use of four full-time counselors was necessary. Counselors were screened carefully in an attempt to match staff with program requirements. It was generally agreed that not all staff members could cope effectively with these difficult to handle youths. Specific selection criteria were: (1) The officer should be capable of maintaining discipline under all conditions; (2) He should be experienced with all aspects of regular institutional duties; (3) He should have participated in the regular officer counselor training program; and (4) He should be highly interested in becoming involved in such a project.

The project began with a two week orientation period for the four counselors. They became acquainted with the purpose of the project, the relevant case history material on all selected boys, and the specific requirements and duties of the counselor positions. After the formal phase of the project began, three meetings per week were scheduled for the purpose of discussing problems, planning specific programs for the week, and collecting opinions and suggestions for immediate and/or future program changes.

The study population consisted of 20 boys. These individuals were selected from the 23 in-resident high P youths. The subjects selected were the most recent 20 admissions who were in the high P category. The three high Ps who were not selected were placed in the contemporary control group along with all high Ps who were admitted to NTS after R.E.A.D.Y. began. A total of 21 different youths were in the control group. During the orientation period initial testing of the experimental subjects was conducted. A graduate student in psychology assisted with data collection and analysis. Testing was repeated periodically throughout the duration of the project for assessment purposes. The counselors filled out questionnaires, rated the boys on several dimensions, and made periodic evaluations of the program.

Structure

Project activities were conducted during the evening hours and on weekends. The 20 subjects lived in their regular cottages and participated in the usual academic and vocational programs. However, instead of the regular evening counseling program, from Monday through Friday the boys were taken to the R.E.A.D.Y. cottage after the evening meal (about 4:45). On weekends they went to the R.E.A.D.Y. cottage at 1:00 p.m. The program ended each evening at 9:00 p.m.

During the time that the project program was operative the

study population boys were separated from the rest of the institution. This permitted a more concentrated effort with the group. It also resulted in a secondary benefit since removing these problem individuals prevented interrupting the program for the rest of the population. For those few activities that could not be held in the program cottage (gym, movies, etc.), the project's subjects were taken as a group to other areas at a time when contact with the rest of the population would be minimized.

The stated purpose of the project, to provide an effective program for the high P individual, necessitated meeting their needs in a highly structured environment. Research indicated that this group craved a great deal of novelty and excitement.[7] R.E.A.D.Y. attempted to provide this. Encouraging physical behavior is contrary to usual institutional programs. On the other hand, *keeping the lid on* does not work with this type of individual. The challenge of R.E.A.D.Y. was to develop the type of environment in which these boys could act out within a structured program while under limits maintained by carefully selected staff personnel. In general, this rationale guided the project program.

Activities

High Ps easily become bored and disinterested in activities. After a period of time at some task, they create their own excitement which usually leads to management problems. One effort made to meet this problem was to avoid long stretches of programming without change. This was accomplished by varying assignment details, in effect splitting half-day assignments of academic and vocational training into four quarter day details.

Getting the cottage cleaned after an evening of R.E.A.D.Y. activity, presented the staff with another type of challenge. They wanted to avoid associating work with punishment. For most of these boys, work already had too many negative connotations. Consequently, the counselors felt they could not assign the clean-up detail to the boy participating the least, nor to the most disruptive individual of the evening.

The solution incorporated the principles behind the R.E.A.D.Y. approach because it was novel, exciting, suspenseful, and effective. A *time bomb* was used. This is a toy which, at the end of the activity each evening, was wound up and passed around among the boys. After a time the bomb made a loud pop. Whoever held the bomb when it exploded was assigned to the clean-up detail. The loser did not *smart talk* the officers, nor did he feel picked on and the R.E.A.D.Y. cottage was maintained in good order.

The exaggerated need for excitement in the high P group leads them to create appropriate diversions when they feel things are getting too dull. Consequently R.E.A.D.Y. strove to meet this need by providing stimulating activity in a controlled environment. Organized games and competitive contests were used as an appropriate outlet for the high P individuals. A chance drawing determined who played what game on any given night. This approach also placed program activity in the hands of the authority figures and most of the students' attempts at manipulation of staff and/or their environment were effectively thwarted.

An example of attempted manipulation was revealed when one of the counselors discovered that the mass bingo games were being rigged. The boys accomplished this by waiting until several had bingo before calling out to the counselor, thus many boys received prizes rather than just one or two. Although this type of cooperative group behavior was conducive to an *esprit de corps* rewarding negative manipulations could not be permitted.

Immediate procedures were taken to introduce a competitive element in the game; i.e., only one per game winner.

Points (one point equals one cent) were used to reward weekly winners of the games determined by accumulative records prominently posted. Additionally, more immediate rewards, nightly bonuses of varying amounts, were awarded by the counselors for appropriate socially approved behavior. There was one bonus per counselor per night. At times special prizes were used with no advance notice for the winners of different contests. These games met with mixed reactions. The boys usually engaged in them wholeheartedly but they verbalized negative feelings about them.

One activity that holds a great deal of interest for most adolescents is auto racing. With points earned in other activities of

R.E.A.D.Y., the youths purchased slot car kits which they assembled themselves. Once they had their own cars they were allowed to run them on a slot car track during specified times. This became a very popular activity for most of the boys. In this instance a chaining of positive consequences for appropriate behavior was established. In order to engage in a highly desirable activity a number of preliminary steps were spelled out. This was one attempt to counter the high Ps' conception of his environment as a haphazard world in which everything depends on luck or getting the breaks and has little to do with one's own behavior.

Psychodrama was initiated to provide a medium of therapeutic exchange among the boys and between staff and inmates. It was selected as an action-oriented therapeutic approach and therefore seemed more appropriate since it avoided the problems, disinterest and general ineffectiveness, of verbal counseling for high P individuals.

It has been stated elsewhere that personnel connected with an institution generally are distrusted by those confined in that facility.[8] Sensing the initial reaction to role playing might be hostile if conducted by regular institutional staff, an outside expert from the psychodrama department of the St. Elizabeth Hospital in Washington, D.C. was hired. Initially, psychodrama was greeted enthusiastically by the boys and there was a great deal of participation. After the introductory period of approximately two weeks, the boys demonstrated a great deal of resistance and hostility toward the activity except for occasional productive sessions. The consensus was that psychodrama did not fulfill expectations of R.E.A.D.Y. program.

Another type of activity which proved to be popular was competitive endeavor with staff. A team of staff members challenged the youths to a softball game. This was received with much enthusiasm and proved to be very successful (the boys won). Although the students also prided themselves on their basketball ability they were shocked to find the staff won this second kind of sports encounter. It was obvious to most observers that team work was more important than physical condition in this game, because the staff had the former but definitely lacked the lat-

ter. The R.E.A.D.Y. boys immediately demanded a rematch which
was accepted. In a hard-fought, well-played game the staff
again won and everybody seemed pleased.

Relations improved decidedly between staff and boys because
of the games but this type of activity requires close control. In
the heat of battle staff members have to be very tolerant because
boys not playing take this opportunity to vent their hostility
verbally toward personnel. With proper preparation and discussion beforehand staff members can deal with this and turn it
into a therapeutic experience for all concerned. Although many
reasons might explain the interest in this type of contest one
strong possibility is the novelty of such active participation by
staff members.

The emphasis throughout the program was on activity, variety,
change and surprise. In keeping with this a novel religious program was initiated. The institution's chaplains engaged
R.E.A.D.Y.'s participants in debates on meaningful controversial
topics. Motion pictures were also used during these once-a-week
sessions to focus on specific problems such as premarital sex, drug
usage, compulsive gambling, lack of involvement with others,
etc. The history of this part of the program was similar to the
role playing. When the youths found a topic that really hit
home interest and participation were high. This occurred spo-
radically, however, resulting in unpredictable group response
from week to week. It may be that active participation should not
be expected every week. Theoretically the high P individuals
lose interest more quickly than others, no matter how stimulating a situation is initially.

Another phase of the R.E.A.D.Y. program was weightlifting
training. This was initiated after a majority of the boys responded overwhelmingly in favor of a demonstration on the topic.
However, a critical error apparently was made in initiating this
program. Instead of telling the youths that this was a new activity they would engage in, the counselors asked who would be interested. Five out of 20 responded positively. Since they had been
approached in this manner, the counselors could not justify requiring them to participate. The remaining 15 boys expressed
their interest by watching the five who did participate.

The experience again demonstrated the failure of verbal persuasion, suggestion, or other similar attempts to reach the high P delinquent. Given a choice or asked their opinion they reacted negatively. Yet when placed in a situation with the necessary equipment and clear guidelines they demonstrated relatively good cooperation and seemed to enjoy what they were doing. This has been evidenced in most phases of the program. For example, the boys responded negatively to questions after special tours, yet they acted enthusiastically while on the trips.

The enthusiasm shown by the youths whenever the staff involved themselves in the activities was evidenced in several areas. Special trips and tours were used occasionally in the project. For example, during a period of two months in the summer, weekly swimming trips were taken to an outside pool. These were enjoyed by most of the youths. However, several felt out of place in the water. One of the counselors, a former lifeguard, began swimming with the boys and offered to teach swimming to the boys interested. This proved to be one of the highlights of the program with several boys becoming fairly good swimmers. The main attraction seemed to be the fact that a counselor was actually in the pool with them.

Control Aspects

In the above discussion it is apparent that these high P individuals were given many opportunities to satisfy their need for excitement. Yet maintaining control at all times was an important aspect of the total project. This was not a volunteer program in which participation was left to the decision of the population. The R.E.A.D.Y. boys were selected because the administrative authorities decided these individuals required more effective programming. Participation for these boys was mandatory. The four correctional officer counselors selected to conduct the program were men who could maintain discipline yet allow the boys to express themselves appropriately. They administered both immediate rewards and prompt controls as needed.

To facilitate the control aspect, two small time out rooms were utilized to provide a negative or punitive contingency following undesirable behavior. The time out rooms have been used with delinquents in other settings with an isolation period of 15 minutes.[9] In the R.E.A.D.Y. project it was felt that extended periods of confinement could lead to the increase in the need for stimulation and consequently more acting out would result from long isolation. Thus a three minute period was selected. During the project the time out room was used a total of 18 times; 11 in the first month, seven in the second month, not at all during the remaining four months.

If an individual's behavior warranted more severe consequences than time out, the regular institutional security unit was used. Only one youth had to be placed in the security unit from the R.E.A.D.Y. cottage. He repeatedly disrupted the scheduled activities and refused to go into the time out room. This was the single failure of the isolation method during a period of six months.

It was felt that the short time out procedure was effective for a number of reasons: (1) It was imposed swiftly following untoward behavior, the negative consequence of surreptitious actions was made clearly apparent to all; (2) it undercut the bravado of going to segregation; (3) it was taking time out from an exciting enjoyable program; (4) it prevented the buildup of tension.

The limit setting in control aspects of R.E.A.D.Y. operated in other ways as well. For example, it was made abundantly clear to all the boys that it was the counselors who decided when activities began and ended. When it was decided that some particular activity ended at 8:30 p.m., that was when it ended, despite grumbles, groans and the fact that the boys were enjoying themselves. The intent here was not to be punitive and deprive the boys of a good time. Rather it was to show them that conformity to rules can result in more good times for everyone. Thus it was imperative to make all aspects of the R.E.A.D.Y. program attractive, to make going along with the authority figures an immediately rewarding experience. In effect the R.E.A.D.Y. program was saying to these difficult to manage youths, "Try it my way and you'll have an even better time than if you do it your way." It taxed the imagination of a very competent staff to make that statement a valid one.

Experimental Design

To ascertain the overall effect of the program the subjects were compared as a group to three kinds of control groups on three different indices of institutional adjustment. One group consisted of previous NTS commitments who would have qualified for the project if there had been one at the time. All the boys in this group were matched with the R.E.A.D.Y. boys on Dr. Quay's personality dimensions, race, IQ, and D.C.—federal commitment. The second control group consisted of boys in the institution at the time of the R.E.A.D.Y. group who were matched with the experimental subjects on the above variables. This contemporary control group was limited in number because of their unauthorized leaving (AWOL). Of 21 boys placed in the contemporary control group, data for comparison were available on only 13 of them. Therefore the most blatant cases were unavailable for comparison with the project group, considerably reducing the possibility of finding statistically significant differences.

The third control group consisted of all boys, both past and contemporary, who were eligible for the R.E.A.D.Y. project. This total control group included all boys in the first two control groups plus any other boys in the same personality grouping and the R.E.A.D.Y. boys who spent at least two months in the institution during the critical six month period. This eliminated those boys who were AWOL or were transferred before two months of the six month period had elapsed. Although this also provides a conservative estimate of differences, it seemed a realistic criteria group. The following indices of institutional adaptation were used to compare project subjects to the three control groups: (1) Average number of days in segregation; (2) Average number of assaultive offenses; and (3) Type of release within the critical six month period.

Findings

The project boys compared to the past control group showed significantly fewer days in the unit—six days compared to 13 days. The difference between the two groups on a number of assaultive offenses while not statistically significant was in the predicted direction, .25 compared to .42 offenses. For type of release positive adjustment was defined as parole within the six month period remaining in the institution; negative adjustment was defined as a disciplinary transfer or an unauthorized leave (elopement) from the institution. A significantly greater proportion of controls showed negative adjustment, 26 percent versus 0 percent. As noted earlier there were few contemporary control cases available for use in the statistical comparison. This is evidence in itself that the R.E.A.D.Y. boys (all of whom did remain for the six months period) adjusted more successfully to the institution than did boys who were eligible but were not selected for the study.

While the differences found were all in the direction of better institutional adjustment for the project group, none of these reached an acceptable level of statistical significance. The R.E.A.D.Y. boys were compared to all eligible control subjects on the three measures of institution adjustment. The project boys averaged significantly fewer days in segregation than the total control group, six days compared to ten days. During the six month program project boys committed a smaller number of assaultive offenses, .25 versus .50 assaultive offenses per boy. Comparison of the number of boys in each group who committed assaultive offenses revealed: 25 percent of the R.E.A.D.Y. boys committed assaultive offenses compared with 33 percent of the controls. This difference, while in the predicted direction, is not statistically significant.

Finally, in comparison to this total control group a greater proportion of project subjects made a positive institutional adjustment, 21 percent compared to 0 percent. In summary all of the comparisons of the R.E.A.D.Y. boys with the various control groups were in the predicted direction, better adjustment and more in-program time for the experimental subjects. While not all of the differences obtained the level of statistical significance it does seem apparent the project group did demonstrate a better level of functioning.

Summary

Project R.E.A.D.Y. demonstrated the efficacy of separating the more *psychopathic* offender from other types of delinquents and using carefully selected staff to control this group, and to treat them. While a number of mistaken assumptions were made in setting up the treatment activities for working with this group, relevant and helpful programs were brought to light. Thus the prime function of project R.E.A.D.Y. was realized. It served as an exploratory endeavor to develop more effective rehabilitative approaches for difficult to manage youth.

In view of the characteristics of this group future program developments should include a willingness to continually reassess the relative effectiveness of program activities. Eventually a catalogue of suitable activities may be developed for dealing with difficult to manage youths. For the present it is clear that this differential treatment approach for the R.E.A.D.Y. type of offender has been effective.

Epilogue

The institution in which this demonstration was conducted closed May 15, 1968, to be replaced by a new one, Edward Kennedy Youth Center, Morgantown, West Virginia. The differential treatment program represents the next developmental step utilizing treatment relevant for the correction of youthful offenders.[10] The answers to questions being explored in this program (what kind of treatment programs, and by what kind of workers, in what kind of settings, are best for what kinds of offenders?) will possibly provide entry into the next phase of correctional management, hopefully bringing about the substitution for the present drawn out, mass managed, intermixed techniques, of shorter, diagnostically appropriate, more effective correctional treatments.

BIBLIOGRAPHY

1. Quay, H. C.: Psychopathic Personality as Pathological Stimulation-Seeking. *American Journal of Psychiatry,* 122:314-325, 1965.
2. Skryzpek, G. J.: The Effect of Perceptual Isolation and Arousal in Anxiety-Complexity Preference and Novelty Preference in Psychopathic and Neurotic Delinquents. Ph.D. Dissertation, University of Illinois, 1966.
3. Orris, J. B.: Visual Monitoring Performance in Three Subgroups of Male Delinquents. M.A. Thesis, University of Illinois, 1967.
4. Quay, H. C., and Levinson, R. B.: The Prediction of Institutional Adjustment of Delinquent Boys, Preliminary Results. Mimeograph, 1966.
5. Quay, H. C., and Peterson, D. R.: The Questionnaire for Measure-

ment of Personality Dimensions Associated with Juvenile Delinquency. Unpublished paper, 1964.

6. Quay, and Levinson: *op. cit.*
7. Orris: *op. cit.*
8. Haskell, M. R.: Group Psychotherapy and Psychodrama in Prison. *Group Psychotherapy,* 13:22-33, 1960.
9. Tyler, V. O., Jr., and Brown, G. D.: The Use of Swift, Brief Isolation as a Group Control Device for Institutional Delinquents. *Behavioral Research and Therapy,* 5:1-9, 1967.
10. Bureau of Prisons: Differential Treatment. . . . A Way to Begin. September, 1970.

Chapter 11

AN ANATOMY OF VIOLENCE

HARRY GIRVETZ, Ph.D.

J OHN HERBES, in his introduction to the report submitted to
the National Commission on the Causes and Prevention of
Violence observed that the commission, as it addressed itself to
the problem of violence in America, was unable to find a significant work on the subject. Although the gap may since have
been at least partly repaired,* H. D. Graham and T. R. Gurr,
editors of the report, found that social scientists "have largely
eschewed the study of violence in America,"[1] and they noted the
absence of an entry on *Violence* in the new edition of the *Encyclopedia of the Social Sciences.*

Writing in 1969, a distinguished scholar, Hannah Arendt, also
found it surprising that violence "has been singled out so seldom
for special consideration"[2] and she went on to find it "a rather
sad reflection on the present state of political science that our
terminology does not distinguish among such key words as *power,
strength, force, authority,* and, finally, *violence.* . . ."[3] I am interested in only two of these terms, *force* and *violence,* and I will
venture definitions somewhat at variance from those on which Dr.
Arendt relies.

Force or violence is harm perpetrated on persons or property
ranging, in the case of persons, from restraining their freedom of
movement to torture and death, and, in the case of property,
from simple fine or damage to complete expropriation or total
destruction. Violence and force are not usually differentiated,
but I find it useful to distinguish them and I think a distinction
can be made without too much defiance of usage.

I would distinguish force by its *legitimacy. Force,* as I here
think of it, is authorized coercion, involving physical or economic sanctions, justified by reference to established principle

---

* For example, see Held, Virginia, *et al.,* (Eds.): *Philosophy and Political
Action.* New York, Oxford University Press, 1972.

and incorporated in a system of law or, in preliterate societies, simply taken for granted as a part of the accepted or traditional *scheme of things*. J. M. Cameron in a recent article on violence rightly points out that "what is taken to be unalterable, a part of the natural order is not singled out as violence."[4] And, of course, what is called force in one culture or period may be regarded as violence in another.

As Cameron notes, brutal floggings which today would be regarded as outrageous and intolerable violence were part of the routine discipline of Wellington's army. But Wellington used *force* to mold his army, not violence. To be sure, there may come a time when the prevailing and heretofore accepted notion of legitimacy is challenged by at least one of the groups in a society whose consent is necessary if there is not to be revolution or civil war. At that point the distinction between force and violence becomes confused until the issue is resolved, as in the case of our Civil War.

It is a distinctive feature of modern social organization that, in contrast to early periods, force is invoked only by the state which is, indeed, accorded a virtual monopoly in its use. If an individual might once have been permitted to punish an assailant, this is no longer the case, although he may, of course, take appropriate emergency measures to protect himself. And, if the church once enjoyed the right to punish heretics, it has long since been bereft of that right. If employers once used private armies to break labor unions (sometimes with appropriate pretense of legitimacy, i.e., government sanction) this could not easily happen in present-day America. Parents may still restrain or punish their children and here and there a teacher may be permitted to use corporal punishment, but such uses of force are peripheral and exercised solely at the discretion of the state.

A common error consists of identifying all exercises of power, particularly when the source is political, with the use or threatened use of force. However, the threat or use of force is far from representing the only way in which the state exercises power. Indeed, the extent to which a government relies on force is a fair index of its weakness. It will rely as much on perquisites: patronage, handouts, and what Americans call *pork*. Above all, it will rely on persuasion, using that term in the broadest sense to include conversion of the major factions or parties in a society to a belief in the fundamentals of the social order of which they are a part, a belief sufficient to provide the kind of basic consensus which assures that opposition is always loyal opposition.

But my theme is violence rather than force and it is to violence, defined as illegitimate and unsanctioned acts of individuals or groups of individuals intended to inflict injury on others, that I wish to give my attention.

It may be said at the outset that the state sometimes uses violence as well as force, that is to say, the coercion it uses may be quite illegitimate, as when the police use coercion punitively and beyond what is needed to quiet a disturbance or restrain a culprit. In Isla Vista, the troubled student community adjoining the campus of the University of California at Santa Barbara, police action was a mixture of force *and* violence. At Mississippi State it was a case of sheer violence. When the state uses its power to coerce for purposes which are extra-legal and have no basis in consent or acknowledged principle, such coercion takes the form of violence. Surely it was violence that the Nazis inflicted on the Jews, violence that Stalin inflicted on his victims, violence that some Southern politicians would inflict on the Negro who rejects their notion of a proper relationship between the races.

However, it does not get us very far to talk about violence in general. It is necessary to distinguish different categories of violence. I find four such categories, although I am not sure that they are exhaustive or mutually exclusive and there may well be a preferable classification.

1. ECONOMIC VIOLENCE. I refer here to the large category in which individuals are driven to violence, that is, to do injury to others, from economic need. I do not include here those hardened criminals for whom satisfying their economic needs in this way has become a way of life which they prefer even though alternative ways of life might be open to them. Neither do I include those who, while their aggressions are directed to an economic reward, cannot be said by prevailing standards to need that reward. On the other hand, the need may not be as exigent as Jean Val-

jean's when he stole a loaf of bread to feed his starving family. I would include the embezzler who steals from his employer to repay gambling debts, the addict who mugs a victim to get money for another *fix*, the recently arrested bankrobber who embarked on his hazardous career because he was hopelessly in debt to loan sharks. Admittedly his was the foolhardy recourse of what we would call a *weak* character.

The point is that neither he, the addict, nor Jean Valjean would have engaged in violence if there had been some other way open to them. Such people would prefer not to be aggressive; the physical harm they do to persons is incidental and often accidental. They have moral standards and are aware of breaching them, even though some of them may be more prone to temptation than the rest of us.

I will not linger on this category, interesting though it may be to ask ourselves whether such crime is on the increase (which I doubt), and what social conditions and methods of correction would reduce such aggression to a minimum. Neither will I raise here the crucial question whether theft is morally justifiable where there is a maldistribution of wealth *that has no functional justification* and the deprived have no other recourse; or where individuals are *arbitrarily* excluded from an opportunity to seek the goods of life. No doubt such arbitrary exclusion explains why Negroes are not convinced that "the laws of theft are as important to Negroes as they are to anyone else," although it so happens that it was a Negro judge, James B. Parsons, the first of his race to be appointed to the federal bench in the continental United States, who said that.

I stress *arbitrary* exclusion. Often the worst disabilities will be tolerated if only a rationale is provided. The commonest rationale is that there isn't enough to go around. A better one is that deprivation endured now will lead to prosperity later. Still another, favored years ago by Calvinists, was that prosperity is a mark of God's favor and poverty of His disfavor. If there is indeed a contempt for law among Negroes, manifest in a far greater incidence among them of economic violence, this will be mitigated only when it becomes evident that they are not gratuitously excluded from the benefits which the law is intended to protect.

2. ANOMIC VIOLENCE. As though nagging poverty were not enough, the island of Sicily, as we all know, is the seat of an infamous society known as the Mafia. Since the families generally referred to by this name often wage relentless war on each other until the ranks of their male members are nearly decimated, the sense in which they may be called a *society* is not altogether unassailable. Nevertheless, the Mafia has its hierarchs and henchmen. Its rulers gather occasionally in formal conference, and it appears to conduct itself by a kind of code, albeit one that is as brutal as it is bizarre.

If we are to believe one of its chroniclers, there was a time when the leaders of the Mafia thought of themselves as social benefactors, although, given the nature of their activities, the claim strains credulity. But whatever the past may have contained, the recent crimes of the Mafia have been so heinous as completely to preclude the possibility that the perpetrators could really believe they were promoting the public good.

This change, if it was one, resulted at least in part from the repatriation of gangsters like the late Lucky Luciano who imparted a certain American efficiency to the antique methods of his more provincial colleagues. Extortion and graft took on new and ingenious forms; traffic in drugs and assorted rackets became a major industry, and violent death a daily occurrence. We are told that the homicide rate of Palermo is the highest in the world, and, since not even the grief-striken relatives of the victims will brave the vengeance of the Mafia by testifying against the murderers, the crimes go unpunished.

The Mafiosi correspond to the anomic men designated by Professor R. M. MacIver as those who have substituted disconnected urges for moral standards. They are a law unto themselves. They rule by terror. Their sole weapon is injury or the threat of injury. They do not pause for preachments, they seek no conversions. Suffering no pangs of conscience, oblivious of the rules by which most men are governed, impervious to considerations of justice, they have no need for those rationalizations, transparent or opaque, by which the normal man tries to conceal his baser motives. They would be the first to scorn ideologues and system-makers; their interests and energies are generally exhausted in the act of pillage itself and the immediate conditions that make it possible. Except as objects of plunder their victims are of only marginal interest to them. It seems appropriate, therefore, to coin the term *mafianism* for all exercises of power that seek no extenuation and have no objective other than plunder, no means other than violence or the threat of violence, and no limit other than the satiation of the oppressor and the impoverishment of his victim.

Happily mafianism is a rare phenomenon, partly because it is a highly inefficient method of exploitation, partly because even the most brutal men generally need some formula for legitimizing their activities. The absence of such a felt need may indeed be taken as pathological and as a hallmark of the truly criminal mind. Thus, mafianism is simply organized criminality—almost institutionalized and in complete control of a society, as under a Duvalier or Trujillo in such blighted Caribbean countries as Haiti and the Dominican Republic, hardly structured and lurking in the interstices of a society as in the case of our own Cosa Nostra.

Social scientists have taken over Durkheim's term *anomie* (or *anomy*) to designate such a state of normlessness. According to R. M. MacIver, "Anomy signifies the state of mind of one who has been pulled up by his moral roots, who no longer has any standards but only disconnected urges, who has no longer any sense of continuity, of folk, of obligation. The anomic man has become spiritually sterile, responsive only to himself, responsible to no one."[5] I would not identify anomic man as thus described with the so-called *psychopathic personality* to be referred to shortly under the title of *psychogenic* violence. Anomic men exhibit what the American Psychiatric Association in its *Manual* on mental disorders calls *dyssocial reaction.* The *Manual* says:

> This term applies to individuals who manifest disregard for the usual social codes, and often come in conflict with them, as a result of having lived all their lives in an abnormal moral environment. They may be capable of strong loyalties. These individuals typically do not show significant personality deviations other than those implied by adherence to the values or code of their own predatory, criminal or other social group.[6]

Harvey Cleckley observes that those showing dyssocial reaction are nonetheless "capable of loyalties and seem in their rebellion against society to have some standards of their own, even though these may be immoral and condemned by law."[7] Tough gangs such as our Hell's Angels or England's Teddy Boys of the 1960's and its present day *skinheads,* may well fall under this rubric.

3. PSYCHOGENIC VIOLENCE. Under this head I include all violence resulting from or associated with mental or personality disorders ranging from psychoneurosis to those major psychiatric disorders which are called psychosis. Included under this rubric is aggression relished or enjoyed for its own sake, which in its more pronounced form is called sadism. Included, also, is the anti-social behavior of psychopaths, a familiar, if baffling, clinical entity. As Cleckley notes, most fully developed psychopaths, in addition to perversely inviting failure in whatever they undertake, "also commit aggressive anti-social acts. They forge checks, swindle, steal repeatedly, lightly indulge in bigamy. . . . Some [commit] murder or other shocking felonies, usually with little or no provocation, often without comprehensible motivation."[8]

And yet the psychopath often exhibits outstanding intellectual ability and, as Cleckley says, is so free from "the manifestations of ordinary psychiatric disorder" that it is difficult to believe that "deep within him may be concealed a deficiency that leads not to conflict or unconscious guilt, but instead makes him incapable of feeling normal remorse or of appreciating adequately the major emotional experiences of human life."[9] Indeed, the psychopath, Cleckley observes, "expresses normal reactions [of love, loyalty, gratitude] with a most impressive appearance of sincerity and depth. . . ."[10]

If psychopaths are at any given moment difficult to identify we must not forget that even in the case of psychotics most clinicians do not distinguish qualitatively between a person suffering from psychosis and so-called normal people. The difference is regarded by them as a quantitative one.* The seemingly most civilized country in Europe taught us in the years preceding and during World War II of the brutal indignities that so-called normal men can inflict upon defenseless victims. We are reminded of this again as we read about the My Lai massacre.

---

* Those who hold that psychotics are qualitatively different see schizophrenia or other *functional* psychoses as having a clear somatic matrix.

I stress this, as I have the psychiatrists' view that the psychotic and normal individual are not different in kind, as I have, also, the deceptive normality under most circumstances of individuals who are actually psychopaths, for special reasons which will become apparent when I turn to my final category of violence, the category that interests me most.

4. IDEOLOGICAL VIOLENCE. I use this term to embrace all violence in behalf of a political or social objective. Here the essential factor is that the individual does not directly promote his own interest or advantage, i.e., that his use of violence serve a *cause*.

I find it useful to distinguish three forms of ideological violence: (a) terrorism (b) insurrection (c) revolution.

(a) TERRORISM. This is a technical term in the lexicon of the political scientist. As the term is used here, terrorism refers to a technique for bringing about social change which relies on the action of heroic, if romantically messianic, individuals, rather than on mass action, and therefore takes the form of sabotage and assassination. Terrorism is never a frontal attack on the police or armed forces but is intended to demoralize the government by destroying strategic targets or striking down specific individuals. Such terrorism is not to be confused with governmental terror which masquerades as law enforcement and is the desperate recourse of rulers so fearful of their tenure that they are bent upon exterminating all real or imagined opponents.

The methods of terrorists are necessarily conspiratorial, and the recourse occurs among those who have either abandoned or never entertained the hope of achieving change by working within the system. Thus the terrorist scorns reform, with its reliance on legal means for effecting social change, as a snare and illusion, even in a democracy. Typical of terrorist groups were the Irish Sinn Feiners, the Russian Socialist Revolutionaries, and the anarchist followers of Bakunin and of Kropotkin with his *Propaganda of the Deed,* and, of course, most recently, the Irish Republican Army. Terrorism was rejected by the Bolsheviks who based their strategy on mass movements and, like Lenin, were hostile to the romantic messianism of the anarchists.

Some of the recent rhetoric of the American New Left could

have been taken verbatim from the 1879 program of the Russian Narodnaya Volya (People's Will):

> Terroristic activity, consisting in destroying the most harmful person in the government, in defending the party against espionage, in punishing the perpetrators of the notable cases of violence and arbitrariness on the part of the administration aims to undermine the prestige of governments' power, to demonstrate steadily the possibility of struggle against the government, to arouse in this manner the revolutionary spirit of the people and their confidence in the success of the cause, and finally, to give shape and direction to the forces fit and trained to carry on the fight.[11]

Terrorists are revolutionists in a hurry, impatient not only with the slow pace of legal reform, even when such reform is available, but with the inertia of the masses whose torch they believe they carry.

Historically, as G. D. H. Cole points out in his *History of Socialist Thought,* terrorism has tended to retard rather than advance the cause of social reform. The victims of the assassins are easily replaced, a regime that might have tolerated dissent or failed out of sheer inefficiency to root out dissent is galvanized into action, and all reformers are more plausibly stigmatized as wild-eyed bomb-throwers.

(b) INSURRECTION, unlike terrorism, is a frontal attack on government, but distinguished from revolution in that it is local in scope, usually limited in aim, and usually deficient in positive program. Generally, the objective in insurrection is modification of government policy. Insurrection would be more appropriately described as rebellion if the objective were territorial secession. Insurrection is common to loosely organized states with a weak national tradition, a weak central government and primitive transportation facilities which reduce the mobility of the government's armed forces.

However, insurrection and its potentialities may require reevaluation in circumstances such as those which prevail in the United States where government can deploy overwhelming force but is reluctant for various reasons to do so. Thus, violent protest may take on an insurrectionary character that it does not ac-

tually have, as in the case of the ghetto riots and the recent riots
on our campuses, where militants are able to capitalize on the
government's reluctance to spread the conflict or the government's
sheer inability to dispense even-handed justice and provide incarceration for small armies of dissidents.

(c) REVOLUTION. Revolutions are of various kinds and I shall
not linger here on an anatomy of revolution. I am concerned
with social revolutions rather than with palace revolutions or
political revolutions although a brief description of the latter is
perhaps in order.

A palace revolution simply rotates the *ins* and *outs* without
significant modification of government policy or disturbance to
the underlying system of class relationships. This has been revolution Latin American style, although one suspects that countries
like Brazil and Argentina are due shortly for another kind of revolution. A political revolution may involve a change in the form
of government, for example, from monarchy to republic, or it
may be an attempt at territorial secession in which case it would
more accurately be termed a rebellion. The revolution of the
American colonies is more aptly called a rebellion. In all such
revolutions the basically prevailing system of privileges and rewards remains intact. It is when these are fundamentally modified that we have a social revolution such as the French Revolution of 1789 or the Bolshevik Revolution of 1917.

It would be tempting at this point to explore in detail the sense
in which the right of revolution is part of our American tradition.
I have done this in my *Evolution of Liberalism* and will not
linger on the topic here. I would rather concentrate on those necessary conditions without which a social revolution cannot occur.
There has been so much loose talk about revolution in our country that we would do well to give these conditions at least brief
attention.

First, a social revolution cannot occur unless there is a fundamental disparity between the power of an ascendant class and the
rights and privileges its members actually enjoy. In the eighteenth
and nineteenth centuries the middle class came increasingly to
possess power. But it lacked the rights and privileges—even

the suffrage—that go along with power. To the question that became the title of his celebrated pamphlet *What Is the Third Estate?* the French Abbé Sieyès answered, "Everything." "What has it been hitherto in the political order?" he asked next. "Nothing," he answered. "What does it desire?" "To be something." A revolution was therefore inevitable.

Second, a social revolution cannot occur unless there is a fundamental disparity between the productive potentialities of a given social system and the extent to which it realizes its potentialities.

In eighteenth century France the prevailing system of class relationships served to retard rather than release the productive capacity of that country. In Marx's terms, which are applicable to the experience of eighteenth century France, as they are to Czarist Russia, there was a contradiction between the *forces of production* and the *relations of production.* That is to say, human and physical and technical resources were available for the expansion of production. But the prevailing socioeconomic system prevented their use. In the 1930's the prevailing system of class relationships that we call capitalism was similarly inhibiting, producing a stagnant condition of mass unemployment and mass deprivation which, had it continued, would surely have led to a revolution.

Even so, it would not have led to a successful revolution in the absence of two more conditions. There must be adequate leadership; and there must be the vision of a way out.

Such are the varieties of violence: economic, anomic, psychogenic, ideological. It is against this background that I would like to discuss the preoccupation, ranging from flirtation to infatuation, of the New Left with violence.

Commenting, before his untimely death, on what he called the rising mystique of violence on the Left, Professor Richard Hofstadter observed: "Those who lived through the rise of European fascism, or who have watched the development of right-wing groups in this country over the last generation, or have fully recognized the amount of violence leveled at civil-rights workers in the South, are never surprised at violence cults on the Right." More arresting, he found, is the decline of commitment to non-violence on the Left, and the growth of a disposition to indulge in or to exalt acts of force or violence.

Let me deal first with the rhetoric.

The far right, says Irving Howe, "shrewder than its symbiotic opposite on the far left, has never articulated an ideology of the rope and the bomb; it has done its dirty business and kept its mouth shut."[12] This is not quite true, to be sure. The Nazi and Fascist glorification of violence for its own sake is too well known to require documentation here. And the philosopher who dreamed that in some other age than this "rotting and introspective present" we may once again have spirits of "sublime malice, spirits rendered potent by wars and victories, to whom conquest, adventure, danger, even pain, have become a need"[13] was hardly a leftist. Thus spoke Nietzsche, echoed by Heidegger who interprets human existence as a "thunderstorm of steel," and preceded by Hegel who found in war the deeper meaning that "by it the ethical health of a nation is preserved." No leftists they.

But Howe is correct about right-wing terrorism in the United States. Our racists and vigilantes, having no intellectual spokesman, have gone about their business in silence. Not so the New Left and such guiding spirits of the New Left as Frantz Fanon. Or Jean Paul Sartre who writes in his introduction to Fanon's *The Wretched of the Earth* that "irrepressible violence . . . is man recreating himself" and that it is through "mad fury" that "the wretched of the Earth" can "become men." Sartre adds that "to shoot down a European is to kill two birds with one stone . . . there remains a dead man and a free man."[14]

However, the rhetoric of violence embraced by the New Left involves more than the elegant articulations of a Sartre or the mystique of a Fanon. It includes the curious use of obscenity, the use of obscenity in contexts where it has never before been used. To be sure, the Left has never been known for its civility. A tradition of verbal abuse goes back at least as far as Marx who is notorious for his acerbity. Leftists are incorrigible schismatics and the language they use in dealing with each other can hardly be called endearing and affectionate. But the vogue of obscenity among leftist militants is something new and different.

Obscenity is not new, of course. It has been part of the common man's language of abuse since there have been common men. No doubt it is his compensation for lacking the vocabulary of the literate and educated. What is *new* is the injection of obscenity into the discourse and debate of literate people in contexts where obscenity has never before been used. This is no longer a continuation of the Marxist tradition of acerbity in debate. Neither should it be understood as an attempt to identify with the common man. It is something else. It is, I contend, an integral part of the New Left's recent preoccupation with violence.

Liberals and libertarians have muted their criticism of the obscenity vogue. No liberal wants to be charged with prudery, nor with being a slave to conventional morality, nor with arbitrarily imposing his standards on others, nor with inhibiting free speech. Criticism of obscenity seems to put one in one or other of these postures. Even worse, no aging liberal wants to be reminded of the generation gap. In consequence, the real point has been obscured and is rarely if ever made. I object to the use of obscenity as a polemical weapon, not because it offends my sensibilities, which it does, but because it halts dialogue and discussion so that no other encounter is possible except a violent one. Beyond this, to characterize an adversary with one or other of the obscenities now in popular use among dissidents is in effect to deprive him of his humanity, to degrade him, to exclude him from the company of decent men.

The import of what one says is that he is beneath contempt; therefore any injury that may be done him is justified. Joe McCarthy's use of the word *Communist* served the same purpose: Communists are disloyal and one does not parley with traitors, one destroys them. Use of *pig* to designate policemen paves the way for the same consequence; after all, pigs are for slaughter. Contrary to the chant we learned as children, words, as well as sticks and stones, *can* break our bones. Obscenity is not innocuous verbal expletive. It is the attempt to inflict pain in circumstances where one lacks the physical means of inflicting injury. The time may have come for us to see that we have been conned, that the obscenity kick is not, and surely not *merely*, an exercise in libertarianism, nor merely a device for mocking authority by saying what is forbidden, nor merely a reflection of our sexual emancipation, nor merely a way of declaring war against middle class values, but an index of our involvement in violence. In the beginning, we might remember, there was the *word*.

Let us now turn from the word to the act. What is the case for violence as we recently heard it made by the New Left?

We are first reminded of the horrors of the Vietnam War. We are confronted with our failure to dispense social justice to our black and brown minorities. We are told of the impoverished one-fifth whose standard of living should indeed affront the conscience of any affluent society. We are reminded of the disgraceful condition of our cities and the neglect of our basic services, of our warped order of priorities, of the enormous gap between our preachment and practice. In my judgment we are justly faulted, although I must add that there is a failure to achieve historical perspective among solipsists who have come to regard the reading of history as irrelevant. To point, for example, to the brutal use of women and children in mines, mills, and sweat-shops at the turn of this century and to note that such exploitation is nearly banished today; to call attention to the reduction of the sixty to sixty-five hour work-week to forty hours is often to evoke wide-eyed surprise from young New Leftists or the charge that one is whitewashing the system. Even so, much of the indictment is deserved. It has, of course, long been voiced by non-violent liberals and leftists.

The conclusion drawn by the militants is that the whole system is hopelessly corrupt. We must tear it down and start over again. It is argued, often, it may be added, with some measure of plausibility, that those in power will reject substantive reform (or pay only lip service to it) unless confronted by violence or the threat of violence. This is the only language they understand. Violence is, after all, very much a part of the American tradition; as American, Rap Brown has told us, as cherry pie. We won our freedom as a nation by recourse to violence and history shows that the great advances of mankind have been made possible by violent revolutions. Anyhow, everything else has been tried and we have no other recourse. Why, indeed, complain about violence; look at what we are doing in Vietnam and what we have done to the black man and the Indian.

I will be brief with those who hope for revolution. None of the conditions for revolution discussed earlier is even remotely present in the United States. On the contrary, majorities and all politically significant minorities in this country oppose each other within the framework of a *basic consensus*. Either implicitly or explicitly, they recognize, underlying their differences, a basic *community of interest* which not only assures a *loyal opposition*, but a tolerant majority prepared to contemplate the possibility of its defeat. Deplorable though it may be, it is a fact that neither the "massed, angered forces of common humanity" nor an ascendant but as yet unrecognized power group is prepared to initiate a substantive change in the prevailing system of class relationships.

The slogan of our Walter Mitty revolutionists, as we all know, is "Power to the People!" Ironically, if the American *people* had their way, left-wing militants would be dealt with as the Russian peasants dealt in the nineteenth century with the Narodniks and they would find themselves in an American equivalent to Siberia. Fortunately, the American people have wisely imposed constitutional restraints on themselves although they express their hostility in other ways: by supporting and electing candidates of the far Right, voting down bond issues for higher education, and calling for more and more suppressive legislation.

Failing in the U.S. to evoke a response from workers, the traditional ally of the Left (at any rate, the kind of response they want—the hooliganism of the hard-hats in New York was, after all, a response), New Leftists have sought a new coalition: of college and university youth, of the poor, and of the minorities.

Now the poor, deplorably numerous though they are—twenty percent in our country—are a hardly formidable army as far as the calculus of power is concerned. That fraction includes the halt and the blind, the superannuated, the incompetent, and a tragic number of children, hardly the stuff of which battalions of insurgents are made.

As for the campus, militants enlist only a fraction of the student body, expanded temporarily when the activist strategists provoke the police into over-reacting. The very fact that such a strategem is regarded as necessary—there is nothing inferential about this, by the way; the strategy has been completely spelled out—the very fact that such a strategem is thought necessary is indicative of the extent to which most students do not share the broader complaints and the deep disillusionment and despair of the radicals. There is widespread discontent.

However, no one really knows the extent to which this discontent is inspired by our participation in a profoundly unpopular war. There is a rejection, concentrated among students in the humanities and social sciences, of what William James once called the *Bitch-goddess, Success,* and a repudiation of the values which have dominated what R. H. Tawney called the *acquisitive* society. However, for the great majority this is hardly comparable to the total alienation and violent hostility which send enragés to the barricades. I would not minimize the political power of the campus. But the campus will not provide many cadres for a revolution.

There remain the ethnic minorities. But the Chicanos and blacks show few signs of cooperating and, in any case, the great majority of blacks do not think in terms of a violent overthrow of the government. A 1969 *Newsweek* poll of Negroes showed sixty-three percent—as against twenty-one percent—who believed they could win their rights without violence. The very militancy of young black intellectuals is proof of progress; militancy does not thrive under conditions of hopelessness. But the same progress that sparks a spirit of revolt in some generates a hope in others that social justice can be achieved within the system.

When Marxists spoke of revolution they had in mind one or other of the great classes that make up a social system. Marx himself would surely have described the dream of New Leftists in the U.S. as sheer adventurism. And, as we all know, the master himself went far astray when he turned to prophecy. The workers of industrialized Europe are uninterested in revolution. The progressive deterioration of their condition that Marx predicted has not come about. And that same system of industrial capitalism which was to lead to their progressive impoverishment has, especially in Britain, the Scandinavian countries and, much more tardily and sluggishly in the U.S., exhibited some capacity for self-reform. New Left militants are, in fact, anachronisms: they have the misfortune to be ideologues in a day when ideology is, if not dead, as some have said, surely in decline. The Social Democrats of Europe prefer to forget Marx and Marxist dogma and to deal with the problems at hand. They are pragmatic rather than doctrinaire. And a similar mood characterizes the major political parties of the United States.

Suppose, however, that the conditions for a revolution *were* present in the United States. Should this be an occasion for self-congratulation? Can anyone who has read about what happened in 1789 or 1917 welcome the blood-letting, the flood of hate, the slaughter of innocent people, the legacy of dictatorship that comes in the wake of these cataclysms? Clearly, some can, some who subscribe, as doctrinaire Marxists mistakenly do, to an iron law of historical progress, whether linear or dialectical, which enables them to believe that something better than what we have now would come of such a bloodbath. For the most part, however, apocalyptic visionaries who preach that the worse things are the better they are speak to shrinking audiences.

There is no danger of revolution in the United States. The real danger is that Americans will over-react to those who phantasize about revolution. To fear that "tiny bands of deracinated intellectuals," as Irving Howe has aptly called them, could wage a revolution is to be as divorced from reality as these would-be revolutionaries. Louis B. Lundborg, board chairman of the Bank of America, perceptively notes the hazard: "I am not afraid the left-wing radicals will win," he observed recently. "I am only afraid of how they will be defeated." He added: "The natural sequel to left-wing radical rebellion is right-wing reaction and repression."

Let us turn from impotent revolutionaries to terrorists. The latter have shown that they do have the power to shut down a great university and virtually incapacitate it. They have shown that they can gut the central section of a city. Their bombs can spread fear even in those great Manhattan temples where the high priests of capitalism normally preside in resplendent comfort and seemingly perfect security. The technique of the terrorist has increasingly beckoned black militants intoxicated with the discovery that they can make the streets of an entire city unsafe after dark and understandably infuriated by the humiliations they daily encounter.

However, violence or the threat of violence will not further the professed cause of terrorists even though temporary concessions may be won. The heavy artillery is commanded by those who oppose their view of social justice or will go only part way. Terrify, alarm a man who commands the artillery and he is likely to use it on you even though he thereby brings about great harm to himself. A frightened man does not act rationally. Arouse his fear and you are lost; your one hope is to appeal to his reason.

Suppose, however, that terrorists are numerous enough to act with impunity. The true idealists among them must ask if they can hope to avoid becoming brutalized by the methods they employ. They must ask if their ends are not fatally compromised by the means used to obtain them. They should, even though they may not, ask themselves if they want to trigger the destructive impulses which, as suggested earlier in the discussion of psychogenic violence, lie latent in the depths of all of us. At what point will they start settling their own notorious differences with the violence they began by directing at others, as the Robespierres and Stalins of history remind us. Not long ago two UCLA black militants were killed on the campus, not lynched by a white mob, that could never happen in California, but by fellow-blacks who had embraced the gospel of militancy and were contesting for leadership.

What assurance have the idealistic militants that the rhetoric some of their comrades use is not a mask for sadists and psychopaths? Earlier, in my discussion of psychogenic violence, I stressed the difficulty encountered in identifying psychopaths, with their deceptive mask of normality. I was thinking of the dilemma in which idealistic militants inevitably find themselves. I am not saying that *they* are psychopaths, although I think that they are often divorced from reality. I am asking how a terrorist can hope to weed out the psychopaths in a kind of undertaking which tends to attract them.

The late Karen Horney, one of the most perceptive writers in the field of psychoanalysis, points out that the compulsive and often fanatical drive to reform others often has sadistic origins springing from the self-loathing of individuals who are unable to measure up to their own idealized image and who externalize their self-contempt by disparaging, humiliating, and ultimately hurting others. Meanwhile they develop a shield of righteousness to protect themselves from their own self-contempt. Some militants should look into Horney's mirror; they may see themselves. Horney's words are worth quoting:

> While he (the sadist) violates the most elementary requirements of human decency, he at the same time harbors within himself an idealized image of particularly high and rigid moral standards. He is one of those . . . who, despairing of ever being able to measure up to such standards, have consciously resolved to be as *bad* as possible. He may succeed in being *bad* and wallow in it with a kind of desperate delight. But by doing so the chasm between the idealized image and the actual self becomes unbridgeable. . . . His self-loathing reaches such dimensions that he cannot take a look at himself. . . . He is compelled, therefore, to externalize his self contempt. . . . He . . . turns his violent contempt for himself outward. Since his righteousness prevents him from seeing his share in any difficulty that arises he must feel that he is the one who is abused and victimized; since he cannot see that the source of all his despair lies within himself he must hold others responsible for it.[15]

I do not say that all or even most militants are sadists, except in the sense that all individuals may have sadistic tendencies. But what are we to think of the militant journalist who declared that "morality comes out of a gun?" What are we to make of the statement of the committee organized to defend three persons charged with the New York City bombings:

> Either the accused did strike a magnificent blow against those who make profit through the destruction of our lives and our world and they are our most courageous and beloved comrades; or they are being framed. . . .

What are we to make of weatherman leader, Bernadine Dohrn's comment on the Sharon Tate murderers, as reported in *The Guardian*, a New Left paper: "Dig it," she said. "First they killed the pigs, then ate dinner in the same room with them, then they even shoved a fork into a victim's stomach! Wild!"[16] These, like the praise some militants had for the assassin of Robert Kennedy, are extreme cases, we may agree. But they are not far from comments recently found in campus newspapers.

Are we to conclude that violence is never justified? Must relief from oppression always await the tardy and usually negligible response of the oppressor? Is violence never effective? It may be agreed that acts of individual violence may sometimes be justified. I would not *morally* condemn the attempt to assassinate Hitler. On the other hand, I might well question the effectiveness of such an attempt.

Where legal or political remedies are available, individual or mass acts of violence are inexcusable, however great the evils against which they are a protest. Political remedies, painfully slow though they may be, are available in a democracy and, if the answer is made that democracy in the U.S. is merely a euphemism for the iron rule of a military-industrial establishment, the plain fact is that the great majority of Americans do not agree. Until they do, recourse to *terrorism* is an admission of lack of popular support. If they do, if the people were to come to the conclusion they were ruled by a dictatorship one might then and only then fall back on Locke's verdict concerning revolution:

> . . . revolutions happen not upon every little mismanagement in public affairs. Great mistakes in the ruling part, many wrong and inconvenient laws, and all the slips of human frailty will be borne by the people without mutiny or murmur. But if a long train of abuses, prevarications and artifices, all tending the same way, make the design visible to the people—and they cannot but feel what they lie under, and see whither they are going—it is not to be wondered that they should then rouse themselves and endeavor to put the rule into such hands which may secure to them the ends for which ancient names and specious forms are so far from being better that they are much worse than the state of nature or pure anarchy. . . .[17]

The weight of Locke's response is even more evident in the following paragraph, which is worth citing in nearly full length. It us one of the most significant passages in the literature of political philosophy.

> Nor let anyone say that mischief can arise from hence as often as it shall please a busy head or turbulent spirit to desire the alteration of the government. It is true such men may stir whenever they

please, but it will be only to their own just ruin and perdition. For till the mischief be grown general, and the ill designs of the rulers become visible, or their attempts sensible to the greater part, the people, who are more disposed to suffer than right themselves by resistance, are not apt to stir. The examples of particular injustice or oppression of here and there an unfortunate man moves them not. But if they universally have a persuasion grounded upon manifest evidence that designs are carrying on against their liberties, and the general course and tendency of things cannot but give them strong suspicions of the evil intention of their governors, who is to be blamed for it? Who can help it if they, who might avoid it, bring themselves into this suspicion? Are the people to be blamed if they have the sense of rational creatures. . . ? And is it not rather their fault who put things in such a posture. . . ?[18]

Revolution can, we may agree with Locke, be *morally* justified. But what of its *effectiveness?* The fatal flaw in the use of violence, revolutionary or other, is, as Hannah Arendt has said, that we can never predict the outcome. To be sure, this handicap applies to all efforts to effect social change, and conservatives stress it in order to discourage all attempts at reform. Why, they characteristically ask, give up a known present for an unknown future? They greatly exaggerate and for the most part they speak more from fear and self-interest than from wisdom.

But their point has genuine applicability to violence as an instrument of social change. The architects of the French and Russian revolutions failed utterly to anticipate the consequences of the great upheavals they set in motion. With all the vast agencies of information and intelligence at their disposal our leaders were unable to predict the outcome of our violent intervention in Vietnam. Too many variables are operative; they consistently baffle the attempts of reason to calculate them. At that point unreason—fear, panic, hysteria, pride ("we have never lost a war")—take over.

And so it is with all violence. That is why our militants increasingly embrace the *cult of spontaneity.* They sense that reason cannot serve them. Given our feeble powers of long-range prediction in human affairs, even where men and groups of men proceed with some measure of rationality, and given the further and profound enfeeblement of these predictive powers when the forces to be calculated are irrational, those who would predict the outcomes of violence are brash indeed. That is why J. M. Cameron concluded, in my judgment with perfect felicity, that if "the consequences of violence are sometimes happy (this) is a grace of fate and not an illustration of the wisdom of the violent."[19]

It is appropriate to conclude with two reminders, one addressed to the militant Left, the other to the alarmed Right. Militant Leftists might well ponder one of Edmund Burke's sagest observations. Commenting on those who habitually engage in criticism and fault-finding, he said: "By hating vice too much they come to love men too little."

Those on the Right who are unnecessarily alarmed and given to overreacting, might be reminded of a fatal flaw in the solution of one of Queen Victoria's possibly less exigent problems. The Crystal Palace, built by Prince Albert, German husband of the Queen, required more than a million square feet of glass. In all it was six hundred yards long and high enough to enclose the trees which dotted the Hyde Park greensward. With the trees birds were enclosed, according to one account, quite accidentally. If intentionally, the systematic German, Albert is said to have designed the palace himself, could hardly have foreseen that the droppings of the birds would mar the valuable exhibits. The birds had to be destroyed. But the use of shotguns in the glass-enclosed structure was out of the question. The Duke of Wellington was called in. True to his reputation, the hero of Spain and Waterloo had a ready solution. "Try sparrow hawks, ma'am," he said.

The historian who tells us this story about the difficulties encountered by the Victorians with their feathered friends neglects to relate how they got rid of the hawks. Before the Right has recourse to hawks it had better solve the problem of how to get rid of them. In the 1930's the German Right failed tragically to solve that problem.

BIBLIOGRAPHY

1. Graham, H. D.: In Gurr, T. R. (Ed.): *The History of Violence in America.* New York, Praeger Publishers, Inc., 1969, p. xxix.
2. Arendt, Hannah: *On Violence.* New York, Harcourt Brace Jovanovich, 1969, p. 8.
3. Arendt: *op. cit.*, p. 43.

4. Cameron, J. M.: Special Supplement: On Violence. *New York Review of Books.* New York, A. Whitney Ellsworth, 15(1):32, July 2, 1970.
5. MacIver, R. M.: *The Ramparts We Guard.* New York, The Macmillan Co., 1950, p. 84. Cf. also Riesman, David: *The Lonely Crowd.* New Haven, Yale University Press, 1950, p. 287ff; and Merton, Robert K.: *Social Theory and Social Structure.* Glencoe, Illinois, The Free Press, 1957, pp. 161-170.
6. *Diagnostic and Statistical Manual, Mental Disorders,* p. 38. Cited by Cleckley, Harvey: Psychopathic Personality. In *Encyclopedia of the Social Sciences,* New York, Macmillan, New ed., Vol. 13, p. 113.
7. Cleckley: *op. cit.*
8. Cleckley: *op. cit.,* p. 114.
9. Cleckley: *op. cit.,* p. 118.
10. Cleckley: *op. cit.,* p. 114.
11. Program of the Executive Committee, 1879: Cf. *Encyclopedia of the Social Sciences,* 1st ed. New York, Macmillan, vol. 14, p. 578.
12. Howe, Irving: Political Terrorism: Hysteria on the Left. *The New York Times Magazine,* April 12, 1970, p. 25.
13. Nietzsche, Friedrich: *The Geneology of Morals.* In Levy, Oscar (Ed.): *Complete Works,* trans., Zimmermann, Helen. New York, Russell and Russell, 1964, p. 24.
14. Sartre, Jean P.: In Fanon, Frantz: *The Wretched of the Earth,* Introduction. New York, Grove Press ed., 1968.
15. Horney, Karen: Our Inner Conflicts. In *The Collected Works of Karen Horney.* New York, W. W. Norton and Co., vol. I, 1937, pp. 203-206.
16. In Howe: *op. cit.,* p. 128.
17. Locke, John: *An Essay Concerning the True, Original, Extent and End of Civil Government.* Oxford, Basil Blackwell and Mott, Ltd., 1946, Ch. 29, par. 225.
18. Locke: *op. cit.,* par. 230.
19. Cameron: *op. cit.,* p. 32.

Chapter 12

PRESENT DILEMMAS AND FUTURE DIRECTIONS OF SOCIAL PSYCHIATRY

PARTICIPANTS: Dr. Norman Q. Brill, moderator; Dr. Price M. Cobbs, Dr. Harry Girvetz, and Burton Kerish.

DR. BRILL: We have covered a broad area during the course of yesterday and today. I am sure there must be many questions you wish to pose and perhaps many comments you wish to make. We've covered subjects such as, Is there anything wrong with youth who tune out? Is there anything wrong with people who burn and kidnap and bomb? To what extent are we ignorant of each other as Dr. Cobbs believes. What is the relationship between war and racism and mental health? What about the need for professionals to take positions and about the admonition that you can't be neutral? What about the need to fight oppression wherever it's found—and I guess that means all over the world? What are some of the details of the program at Lompoc? What about the whole question of violence and obscenities? If you have comments or questions please direct them to a specific individual and we'll just proceed from there. I'll act as the moderator and recognize the hands as they come up.

QUESTION: Dr. Cobbs, I'd like you to compare, if possible, the leadership of the black community. Which of the two different factions, the one led by Whitney Young and Martin Luther King or the one led by Cleaver and Rap Brown, is going to be more effective in getting for the black people an equal position in society? Secondly, what influence do you feel did ghetto opium addiction during the last twenty or thirty years exercise upon our white middle-class kids' drug problems today?

DR. COBBS: After the book *Black Rage* appeared we went on tours and lectures and I found myself answering questions on which I really had no authority. Because of my background as a physician, as a psychiatrist, I certainly have studied a great many social situations. In regard to a comparison of Whitney Young,

200

Martin Luther King, Jr., Eldridge Cleaver and Rap Brown, I cannot give anybody other than an *off the top of my head* opinion. Like most of us, I have no particular reluctance to do it but I don't see it as particularly enlightening.

As to the question of opium addiction, opiates, and their history in the black community, I can tell you a great deal. Drugs in the black community have never been far from most of us. There is a record by Bessie Smith (I think cut in 1928 or 1929) in which she talks about reefers. Most of us who grew up in black communities were very aware of grass as quite young kids. And psychologically it always was an escape, and here I am talking psychologically, from what a person felt as an oppressive reality.

When the Haight-Ashbury first started and you ran into large numbers of young white adults on drugs, psychologically they followed often a different direction. They saw the drug experience as freeing. They saw it as giving unity to a relatively fragmented life. If we were to look at groups of black youngsters and groups of white youngsters the psychological etiology probably would be dissimilar rather than similar.

Certainly, some of the white protest youth now identify with the psychological motivation of blacks, for as they look at the system, they, too, feel excluded and alienated, if that's the word. But as we get deeper into the problem I think the analogies stop. The white youngsters, it would appear to me, psychologically are trying to escape from a different set of shackles, a much more personal set of shackles than the black youngster. The black youngster's shackles seem to be primarily sociological rather than psychological.

QUESTION: Dr. Girvetz, you have always been regarded as a rebel on the campus; yet when during the Isla Vista disturbances you said that "if you call a policeman PIG for long enough, he will start acting like a pig," you were regarded as a staunch conservative. I do not think you have changed your opinions for I have known you as a liberal for many years and you did not change your opinions during this time. But could you comment if the change of times has made you more of a pessimist. I feel optimistic about the future but I felt in your paper a note of pessimism. Could you comment on that?

DR. GIRVETZ: Well, this is a rather personal question and I don't want to weary you with autobiographical detail. I certainly am not a pessimist. I define a pessimist as one who believes that it's a good wind that blows no ill. I have never subscribed to that belief. In case that doesn't move you, I also define a pessimist as someone who believes that every silver lining has a cloud, and I have never subscribed to that either. I am really an optimist.

It is true that in militant new left circles I am regarded as a conservative. I think it rather confuses their taxonomy when I happen to be the one who initiates campaign drives for the support of the lettuce strikers in Salinas and for full page ads in our paper protesting our criminal involvement in an unjust war and so on. But presumably one is a conservative if he says the kind of thing that I have just now said and if he calls attention to the fact that reformers are more interested in getting emotional release by doing their thing rather than by realizing important social goals. My eye is fixed on the goal. That is what I want to get. And when people indulging themselves jeopardize that goal, I intend to tell them so even though they accuse me of the heinous crime of being a conservative.

DR. COBBS: The conservative-liberal labels, I think, don't have much accuracy in today's world. I'd rather focus on the literate man. Dr. Girvetz, during your talk you mentioned the literate man and I wonder if the literate man does not have an obligation to understand the etiology of obscenity rather than to respond to the word and the symptom.

Earlier we were talking about a widening conception of America. As we broaden our heretofore narrow experience and begin to understand more about the various cultures we may come to see that what is obscene to one man may be completely acceptable to someone else. And to me the literate man in today's world has an obligation to go past what is considered obscenity and get to the etiology of it. This would be a quarrel that I would have with you—not whether one is conservative or liberal—but how far one's literateness goes.

DR. GIRVETZ: I am interested in the etiology of obscenity, in its causes. I quite agree with Dr. Cobbs that the scholar has a responsibility to explore both. However, I think it's possible to go too far in the direction of relativism, a relativism which might culminate in precisely the kind of moral skepticism, Dr. Cobbs, that would defeat the moral objectives that you and I share. Your talk was a moral preachment and I believe in such moral preachments. But it's impossible to make an appeal to moral standards without assuming that there are such standards. And that assumption is vitiated by a complete relativism. The fact that some people do something and do it as a group doesn't necessarily establish it, cultural relativists notwithstanding, as morally right.

I suggest two reasons for obscenity being morally wrong. One reason is that it is prelude to violence. And the other reason is that it interrupts and breaks down dialogue, the purpose of which is to effect conversion to precisely the kind of social justice, including racial justice, that you espouse. That's why I object to obscenity. In certain areas and with certain groups obscenity is more natural than with other groups. And clearly it's more natural with people who are uneducated and people who have had no contact with any other kind of discourse.

I actually was not addressing myself to that use of obscenity which is commonplace and with which we have always lived. What I am addressing myself to is the kind of obscenity that has invaded the discourse of educated people, that has corrupted the classroom when permissive teachers allow it. I don't intend to be such a permissive teacher. When anyone engages in obscenity in my class, he will be invited to leave.

COMMENT: Dr. Girvetz, I believe your definition of violence broke down as you progressed when you lost sight of the whole context of the word violence and increasingly focused on active violence of guns. You didn't give much thought to or analysis of the violence that spawned at least one black group you referred to. I think your arguments suspect because your interpretation of the war between the BSU group and the Panthers at UCLA was between one group that believes in violence, in the power of the gun, and another group, the cultural nationalists, who believe justice for blacks can be won through Swahili and cultural exchange. It was not one black violent group against another black violent group.

DR. GIRVETZ: I did not say that two violent groups were involved. I really don't know. I do know that two blacks were killed by other blacks. And I do know that killings like these become easier when there has been a constant flirtation with violence. Then it becomes easier to deploy violence against one's own kind, as easy as against the enemy. The symbols of violence finally turning on one's own kind on a massive scale are Stalin's executions of old Bolsheviks.

As for my record in deploring economic and social violence in society at large I really don't have to defend myself on that. I would much rather have spent my time here dwelling on the sickness of our society than on our left-wing Cassandras. But there are all too few people of my kind who deal with the new left and their violence, and people of my kind should speak out against it.

QUESTION: Did you say that you would chuck a student out who uses profane words? How do you justify forcing a student out who comes from a ghetto where these words are acceptable? As an educated person should you not know that some words are acceptable in the ghetto that are not acceptable among the educated? How do you justify breaking down the dialogue by your chucking that student out?

DR. GIRVETZ: I've never had that experience.

DR. COBBS: I have and I agree, it's a very important point. I might, by a given patient, by a given group, be called all kinds of things. If you are involved with groups on your campus I would not doubt that you would be called all kinds of things, starting with *Honky* and going on from there. But, if you talk to people with whom you ought to continue the dialogue, the onus is on you as the literate man to get beyond cultural barriers and to continue the dialogue. To me, this is the essence of therapy, the essence of education. And I think by trying to define it that way no one is condoning a student's coming into Dr. Girvetz' office and cussing him out.

QUESTION: Dr. Cobbs, in reading your book *Black Rage* as well as another recent book *Graffitti—the Message of Obscenity,* I found a more meaningful example of obscenity than those of Dr. Girvetz. You describe the display of wares in television commercials, of foods which the average black child does not see on his table for a whole year. He gets a barrage of such commercials every five minutes, everyday, and now even in color. What alternatives do we have in educating the public to an awareness of that obscenity?

DR. COBBS: Yes, I think it's a very important question. We—Bill Grier and I—analyzed this problem in trying to understand the Watts riots. Why Watts rather than some place else? Having grown up in Los Angeles I had the feeling that there was some connection between blacks rioting in Los Angeles and Hollywood's television. Many of the journalists who came out from the East to see Watts said, "Now this doesn't look like Harlem, this doesn't look like South Side Chicago." You see, the five minute commercials which dominate Southern California more than other parts of the country contain an ethic of quick and easy abundance, a type of materialism which accentuates what one doesn't have. This had built up a great degree of frustration.

To me it was very significant that this first riot occurred at a time when the first group of black youngsters who were raised on a steady diet of television had attained adolescence. Having seen daily in five-minute doses the unreality of their own particular world, namely that they were not driving the kinds of cars, the symbols of affluence, they saw on the screen, they erupted in rage at a given point. The solutions, I think, have been suggested by any number of people. For one, we should try to understand racism in terms of the national character, in terms of our institutions. For another we should push programs faster and attempt any number of economic alternatives about which other people would know much more than I do.

QUESTION: It strikes me that education and language create barriers between people in a society, of the educated versus the uneducated. The person who receives an education or who acquires language skills sets himself apart from those portions of humanity who do not have this privilege. Do such barriers of language really exist and if so, what should we do about them?

DR. COBBS: I think they do. This came out very strongly during the 1960's in terms of the black movement. The question then was, if we have ten or fifteen percent educated blacks, are they inherently and permanently split off from their fellows who are not educated? I believe that people such as myself have the obligation of broadening their knowledge about a different experience, so that their language encompasses the language used by the other ninety percent.

As Dr. Girvetz talked, I was thinking about the *dozens*. I'm certain you don't know the *dozens* (I see the brother back there grinning, he knows the dozens). The dozens is a form of verbal abuse young black fellows indulge in. If we were to engage in the dozens it would be the most obscene thing you people have heard. It's very much a part of the culture I grew up with. Well, if I, as an educated man, cut myself off from my past it might prevent me from relating to a twelve or thirteen-year-old kid who is not being obscene, who is responding from his culture.

To me, having an education means that one encompasses as many different backgrounds as possible so that education broadens one rather than separates him from those people who don't have an education. I think any teacher, any therapist, who sees people who are uneducated, should not develop some kind of pseudo-language but rather broaden his usage by learning what words mean to his clients, by how they're used, by what the phrases are, by what the nuances are so that they understand him and are able to communicate with him.

In some schools I know in Berkeley, a teacher, a principal, is setting up a course in English as a second language. When I first heard it I thought it was gimmicky but the more I talked to him, the more I was convinced it was very sound. For the black child who learns correct English usage in such a course is not picking up something labelled either superior or inferior, but rather something different from his own language. He is merely broadening his way of expressing things.

DR. GIRVETZ: The area of the uses of language is a bewilderingly complex one. Language can be used for purposes of display; it can be used for purposes of establishing invidious differences; it can be used to bring about understanding. Language is a supple, versatile instrument and unless one learns the kind of uses of it that prevail on a university campus, he hasn't made available to himself one of the most marvelous instruments that we have for communicating difficult ideas.

Now there is a special problem, as you well point out, that is, when one is dealing with students who have not been exposed to one kind of English. I don't pretend to know how that problem can be solved on a university campus. But I do know this: I don't intend to relate to my students by talking to them in monosyllables. I intend to bring them up to the language, to the level of the language employed by informed, educated people.

QUESTION: Mr. Kerish, how do you suggest improving our correctional institutions?

MR. KERISH: The development of a correctional institution, although the institution was begun for different reasons, parallels the development of mental hospitals. How old is our present penitentiary system? It was initiated by the Quakers in Pennsylvania, and those who were locked up were debtors and those awaiting trial. Punishment was physical and followed swiftly after the trial. Now we lock up everybody who violates the law, anyone who frightens someone else. What Dr. Bierer said yesterday about dangerous patients applies with the same ratios to prison inmates. There are just not that many dangerous people around. We just have to educate people that the dangers are not that great, that we do not need to lock up offenders. If we removed the public's fears we can manage offenders in halfway houses, in day-care centers or through probation and parole.

DR. BRILL: I was talking about that very subject with a consultant to a state prison who painted a somewhat different picture about the danger. I wonder if he would care to say a few words about that . . . just to round out the picture.

CONSULTANT: I think that the parallel between the mental hospital system and the prison system is a good one. The only trouble is that the skills have not yet been developed to handle the type of inmate we have in the prisons. Those skills have not been developed well enough to begin to phase out the correctional facility. The state hospital system developed because we knew no other way to handle the mentally ill. When the skills were developed to treat mental patients outside the hospitals, we could afford to shut the state hospitals down. I think the same thing is going to happen with the prison system. When we really understand how to treat the socially destructive person we will close correctional facilities. But at present there are a very significant number of destructive persons, as a matter of fact, there are in this state five hundred people who are so dangerous that scarcely two of them can be let out together at one time.

You people have no concept of what the people in the prisons are like and that's unfortunate, you should. The mental health movement made sure that you found out what was happening in the mental institutions. Now you have to find out what's really going on in prisons and what kind of people are there. They are dangerous, tremendously dangerous. Usually to one another. My institution has been open since about 1950 and during that time we had lost no staff member until a year or two ago. Now we have lost three. But we annually lose five or six to a dozen inmates from assaults of other inmates.

The big problem in a prison is generally the safety of the inmates; it isn't the safety of the staff. So, what is going to happen if we phase out the state prison? Most of us wonder sometimes and I am not a person who says lock them up, but we wonder sometimes why people are put out on parole or on probation or are even allowed to go on bail when we can predict with a hundred percent accuracy that they are going to commit another felony before they are brought to trial.

MR. KERISH: Not only do we predict it, we engineer it.

CONSULTANT: No we don't engineer it.

MR. KERISH: Yes, we do.

DR. COBBS: It seems to me your analysis is superficial. I, like Dr. Girvetz, feel that one has to take some view of history. When I was a consultant at a prison I can recall the time when the Black Muslims were very big in prisons and the Department of Corrections spent a great deal of effort in trying to keep their literature out. That was when they still were nonviolent in terms of their credos. I think that the repressive attitudes expressed then have something to do with the violence now. I would think that there was an interaction between the inmate and the correctional system, between the inmate and society. In any kind of interaction many factors are involved. One would have to consider these many factors in any kind of prediction as to whether or not a felony would be committed when the prisoner got out. I think professionals should not indulge in irresponsible speculation why or when a felon may commit a crime. I don't think we can predict until we achieve a greater depth of analysis.

Dr. Kerish: I am sure it sounds to the audience as if the men at other state institutions are different from the men at Lompoc. I submit that they are not. We have men at Lompoc who have been at Soledad. We have men at Lompoc who have been at San Quentin. And quite the same things happen at San Quentin that happen at Soledad. In the ten years I have been at Lompoc we have had two killings. Now that's a damn sight better ratio than you have in the City of Santa Barbara. And our men are jammed in, not jammed in as badly as at other institutions, and I think that's part of it. But it's the attitudes of the institutions that are different. And I submit that I can take two of your men whom you can't let out together and put them in the population at Lompoc. And they are not going to kill each other. And I don't think I have to go into detail as to why. The reasons aren't there. It's the suppression in institutions such as Soledad and such as San Quentin that engineer that behavior. It's the suppression of society, of the parolee and the probationer that contribute to felonious behavior.

Consultant: I am not acquainted with what's happened at your institution, I only know vaguely that you have a younger group of inmates. But by our very benevolence we have created a problem at San Quentin and at Soledad and the Folsom Institution. In this state in the last fifteen years no medium or close-custody institutions have been built. Every new institution has been a minimum-custody institution. We want to move in this direction, but what does this mean? Only those prisoners are left at the few close-custody institutions who cannot handle a minimum custody institution.

Question: I think the differences between San Quentin prison and Lompoc prison Mr. Kerish mentioned is interesting and important. The problem of environmental design Mr. Rozenfeld brought up yesterday seems to be of primary importance in regard to these two institutions. The difference in environment and in attitude between those two institutions would allow you to do different things at Lompoc than you can do at San Quentin. Now the selecting-out process that was mentioned in regard to maximum security institutions suggests that we have hardened criminals in those institutions while we have curable inmates at minimum security institutions. Yet the warden at San Quentin maintains that the problem of racism is of utmost importance in dealing with the inmates in his institution. Now, my question would be to both Dr. Cobbs and to Mr. Kerish. How do the two factors, racism and the selecting-out of some prisoner as curable, relate to one another?

DR. COBBS: I will certainly let Mr. Kerish say something about Lompoc and San Quentin. I think if I described the Warsaw Ghetto in the manner given earlier,* I would hope that Mr. Kerish would call me intellectually shoddy so that I would try to find out what a ghetto was, how it was created. All too often we ascribe psychopathology to an individual when we are talking about the psychopathology of a society. So *intellectually shoddy* to me is not a label. I use the words to point out that we have an obligation to at least try to be as accurate as possible. I certainly listened to what Dr. Girvetz was saying, he was making one point and wanted to make that clear but he was aware that there were other points that he did not mention. I think if one talks about prisons and a particular kind of selection process and if a particular group is overrepresented at that prison, then one has some obligation to find out why that is so. Is it that all the dangerous criminals are black and brown? And I suggest that by some selection process they are very much over-represented in any prison. One has some obligation to take a look into one's field, into the so-called psychopathology of that individual and his interaction with the psychopathology of that society. Without doing that I think we aren't talking to each other, we are just using epithets.

DR. BRILL: Dr. Bierer, you wanted to say something.

DR. BIERER: I'd just like to put a question. The more we lock people up, the more violence we have in mental hospital facilities and prisons. The more billions you spend and give as charity

---

* This comment refers to a definition of *ghetto* given by a member of the audience.

to various nations, the more they hate you. How can you find answers to these questions, to the question of schooling, of revolution, of poverty whilst giving away these billions. Why aren't you doing anything about that?

DR. BRILL: Would anyone wish to respond?

DR. CARLETON: In answer to Dr. Bierer's question, I should like to emphasize that he, probably most of us here, and a small percentage of other people and professionals actually believe there is much need for change in the methods of treatment of the emotionally ill. Until more people become better educated and develop different attitudes constructive change will come slowly. Further, most people do not care enough about the problem to make the effort to effect improvement. Let me be quick to add, however, that we have, and that we are, experiencing great changes in this country and in this state in particular in our treatment orientation and practices. We are closing down large state mental hospitals. We are treating people as human beings and employing some of the innovations which you, Dr. Bierer, have originated. These include day hospitalization, self-governing units, and other social psychiatric methods.

We can and are looking for the answers to your questions in many areas. The multidisciplinary approach appears to be the most effective orientation to use. This workshop was specifically designed to bring together a group of speakers and to urge audience participation from a number of different disciplines and orientations that we might put our heads together, so to speak, and learn from each other. We need to expose ourselves to critical evaluations of the very cores of our beings, our value systems, our religious myths and our legal myths. These so-called foundations of our civilization may be contributing to our problems. Changes in these areas are very painful. Even some professionals deliberately strive for mediocrity, having gained their degrees, credentials, and having established themselves in relatively comfortable nitches, they fight hard to resist change and hold back improvements.

Realistically, changes come slowly but some of us must push forward the frontiers and explore the unknown. That is the task of this workshop. We are seeking and developing new methods of evolving social, medical and intellectual growth.

I believe your question speaks to the heart of the matter, Dr. Bierer, and I hope others will respond and contribute their answers also.

JUDGE LODGE: I'm Joe Lodge, and I am a presiding judge of the local Municipal Courts in the Santa Barbara area. There are two comments I would like to make about the incidence of violence in the prisons. I think that those of us on the outside are very concerned with what goes on there and are threatened by it. I also would disagree with the consultant to the state prison system. Sometimes I feel very threatened and think there is much violence around. But working with a number of criminals over a period of years I tend to end up with Mr. Kerish. Let me just give you two examples that might be helpful.

In the last month I was asked by a group of felons in the county to meet with them because they wanted to rake a judge over the coals and they asked if I would come. They knew of me and thought I might come. They were all on parole and the parole officer conveyed the request. He said, "Let me tell you, however, they're all felons." And he said, "This is a group of our hardcore felons." Then he added, "You might find it unpleasant and you don't need to feel you have to come." I went. We had a very interesting evening. I didn't know what any of these people were charged with until after the evening when I went over it with the parole officer. And I said, "Tell me about these men, what goes on? It didn't really seem so bad. This one fellow, what was he charged with?" "Well, he was charged with selling pornography in town, not to kids, but to adults." The majority of the rest of them, of these hard-core felons, were on marijuana charges.

The second example I think helpful, I will conclude with. Atascadero has been mentioned earlier. For those of you who don't know, Atascadero is the state hospital prison where we send almost all of the criminally insane (a legal designation), and almost all of the aggravated sexual offenders from the southern part of the state. These are all people whom professionals in one way or another fear. You know, I have seen and dealt with many murderers and I am like any of you when I see one come in, even if it's a young kid and even if I know he's not going to murder again I am sort of scared. Anybody who has the label *criminally insane* attached to them makes you want to look at him, you want to see—well who is he? Is he an animal, is he like us, what have we here?

And with violent people and especially those who, as Dr. Cobbs suggests, come from different cultures, from different ways of understanding and expressing themselves, it is important to me, being in a judging situation, to have contact, to be able to analyze out my own fears. In dealing with and sentencing somebody, either as a psychiatrist sentencing a man to a hospital or a judge sentencing a man to a prison, we need to have enough contact with the allegedly violent people so that we are able to separate out our own fears and then hopefully be able to deal objectively with the person before us. In any event, to maintain contact I think judges should go into these institutions.

The example I'm getting to is that last year Atascadero did a marvelous thing. They set up a judicial day that would be devoted to the judges of the southern part of the state which Atascadero serves. Some five or six hundred of us were invited because there are that many municipal and superior court judges in the southern part of this state. We were free to do pretty much as we wanted. The event started at about seven or eight in the morning and went into the evening. We could eat with inmates without worrying about having guards or even staff with us. We could go into any dorms. We could sit in on any therapy sessions; we could find out what we wanted to, and there are some marvelous programs going on up there.

The inmates have a great deal of control in the institution; it's the kind of thing I think Dr. Bierer would be proud of. I came away from there most enthused, walking on air. Most of these inmates were delighted with what was going on there. Person after person would come up to me, the kind of person whom you fear, you would edge back from as a judge. And you think, "What am I edging back from, I've got to get into this and see where I am and come up with something fair." Now I remember one man who raped his own daughter (and this was not a step-parent rape which is fairly common), it was his own daughter. I remember him saying that, until he had gotten into this institution, he had gone for twelve years without really talking to anybody. He ran a gasoline station, so he was up from about 6:30 in the morning until late at night. He rarely talked to his wife and things finally just broke. He had no friends at that time. Well, he suddenly became a human being to me.

I only go through this example to tell you the one closing point and then I'll leave you. *I was the only judge in this state who attended!* We are the people who know about sentencing. We are the people who are supposed to go in and wade in and get through our own fears and understand the people who are allegedly violent. Or get to understand the blacks, which is another thing. I have the same problem as everyone of you, I'm obviously not black, and I'm scared when I meet the different words and when I really don't know their meaning, when it is a different expression. To be frank about it I get scared a lot of the time, and I find the best way to get over it is to wade in and get close enough so I can see who the people are. But what I have never gotten over, and I hope in a sense you'll never get over, is the fact that it's too bad if we professionals shy away from contact to the point that only *one judge shows up.*

PART V
NATIONS AND COMMUNITIES:
TOWARD A HEALTHY WORLD

Chapter 13

IDENTITY AND VIOLENCE:
IN PURSUIT OF THE CAUSES OF WAR
AND ORGANIZED VIOLENCE*

LOUIS MILLER, M.D.

I WILL NOT DISCUSS particularly the sources and nature of individual aggression however it may provide the motive power for all forms of violence. I will seek the causes of organized
group violence in factors specific to the group itself. I will not be
able to analyze comparatively the problems of the antagonist
groups in any particular situation of group conflict but must
confine myself to a consideration of the general issues in our group
culture which make for war.

My aim will be the pursuit of a particularly profound and tena-
cious group source of war. This source of war is in the very nature of our group culture itself and of our identification with it.
It is in the essence of group identity and self-esteem to be particularly sensitive, proud and insecure, and to react with violence to threat and insult. Group culture is designed to control
in-group aggression but it does this frequently by permitting or
even promoting aggression against other groups.[1]

My submission will be therefore that war and organized violence are at once a result of the nature of group acculturation
and of its product—group identity. In the present dispensation of
things and in history group culture, group identity and group
aggression are one. It is therefore in the group processes that
one should seek the causes and the prevention of war.

Many theses have been developed to explain the phenomena of
organized human violence both in its civil forms and in its full
military dress. These theses explain war and organized violence:
(1) as reactions to a threat, real or phantasized, to the survival
of groups; (2) as expressions of economic appetites; (3) as re-

---

* Presented at the Fifth World Congress of Psychiatry, Mexico City, November,
1971.

217

sults of frustration, unsatisfied sexual needs and other individual psychological problems translated into a group psychology; (4) as expressions of the residues of inborn individual aggression in spite of its acculturation by civilization; (5) as products of individual and group power motives and those of domination; (6) as the result of boredom with the peaceful existence of the group; (7) as a result of an education for violence and war and their elevation to a positive value; (8) as xenophobic reactions; (9) as hereditary impulses and temperamental weakness.

Most of these rationales do or may have something to do with particular instances of group violence and war. On the whole I do not believe that they are fundamental, nor do they supply a general explanation which must be sought for so general and historic a phenomenon.

One may postulate the following about human aggression:

1. Man is born with individual aggressive drives, no less than animals.[2,3] However one cannot ascribe to man a group aggression (herd) instinct as Lorenz seems to do.[4]

2. Individual aggressive reactions are elicited through frustration of instinct.[5] Beyond the frustration hypothesis, I add, that aggression is probably primitively liberated in animals and man where there is a perceived threat to life.

3. I agree with Lorenz that individual man, unlike other animals, has no inborn, autonomic, control mechanisms for his aggression. (Play in man, however, may be a rudimentary innate control of aggression.)

4. Man as an individual has the potential to develop, through acculturation, complex control mechanisms, which become inextricably linked to the cultural control patterns of the group. Thus the control of individual aggression is the result of individual acculturation by the group and control becomes a function of the group as well as of the individual.

5. Man is able to develop the highest forms of the control of aggression which at times seem to border on the autonomic but are capable of change when he is outside of the group or liable to deterioration. The controls are different in type or degree in different cultures to which they are linked.

6. Aggression in man therefore is not primarily a group-linked

drive, as it may be with some animals. As individual human controls of aggression are developed and maintained by the group (group linked and oriented) so the conditions for and modes of expression of individual aggression in man are developed by the group and therefore become group oriented and linked. Thus man is acculturated not only to group control of aggression but to group expressions of aggression such as in war and organized violence.

Freud has remarked upon le Bon's description of crowd reactions.[6] The individual in the crowd tends to feel and react as the crowd dictates and to suspend judgment before its impulses.

Freud writes with some esteem of le Bon's analysis of the effects of the crowd on the individual and his ego. Freud cannot accept le Bon's view that the crowd's behavior is spontaneous and that the crowd arises *de novo*. Cultural antecedents are at work. Freud therefore has no need to fall back on a group or herd instinct. Group feelings arise through acculturation of relations of the individual ego-ideal to the leader. This is an example of a pattern, which arising through acculturation I have called group-linked and group-oriented. Freud subscribes to le Bon's thesis of crowd susceptibility to suggestion. Crowds, Freud says, are either hypnotized by themselves or by their leaders.

Le Bon's thesis on crowds does not however seem useful to explain organized warfare. And Freud's description of the acculturated group hypnotized by the leader stops short before the issue of war which he does not discuss in this context. (Later Freud was to feel that war is the result of a failure of the acculturation of aggression.) In any case, to me crowds seem more nearly allied to the mass than to the group and neither crowd nor the mass phenomena seem to have much to contribute to the understanding of organized group aggression and war. We will finally have to think in terms of much more organized group behavior.

To le Bon's picture of the hypnotized crowd as an example of the mass impress we should add an even more regressive phenomenon of extreme crowd behavior. These extremes demonstrate adequately that man is *not* fundamentally an animal of the group. The phenomena to which I refer are those of mass reactions of the most primitive quality, panic, carnage and orgy. In these totally regressive reactions man is no more related to the group except as an environment quite distinct from himself. He regresses in the stampede to an individual concerned only with his own survival. The *group* for him is only a source of signals about his own possibilities for survival or merely a threat to his own individual survival needs.

The same picture holds for carnage *en-masse,* man is here purely involved with the acting out of his own desire to kill. Here too he is essentially unrelated to those around him. Orgy is an equally egocentric acting out of instinct. This individual-*en-masse* reaction may not be absent in the so called epidemic of drug taking of our own day.

The phases of the suspension of the social bonds and of guilt and shame in the mass and the contagion of the particular instinctual act are not the subject now of my interest, nor is the return of group controls after catharsis. Warfare is not at all related to such profound regressions but these situations do show of what individually oriented drives aggressive man is basically composed, before his acculturation by the group.

I have said that although acculturation in the group produces group-linked controls of aggression its group-linked aggression tends to be turned against other groups. The obverse of acculturation in the group is thus frequently seen as aggression against other groups (out-groups). It is to acculturation rather than to a herd instinct that one must appeal to explain aggression against the out-group.

War therefore is not to be explained as a hypnotic crowd reaction. It is also certainly not a regressive mass phenomenon. War is the product of innate individual aggression acculturated as group readiness to be turned against strange groups. We may thus speak of a culture of war and organized violence.

The compulsive cycles of war between large ethnic and political groups are group events profoundly organized, with a very limited quantity of personal catharsis or of direct individual instinctual satisfaction (as opposed to the case of mass phenomena). Wars are organized on a very high personal psychological and group level. True, in wars, there is great selectivity of the objects to which the social values are directed but values remain essentially operative. There is, of course, a devaluation of the *enemy* group but the evaluation of the in-group rises to ideal and sometimes religious heights. Wars are involved often with great personal sacrifice for the common good. The new forms sanctioned for aggression are strictly group determined and outwardly directed. This too relates to my contention that war is a cultural state.

Further, mass and crowd reactions do not resemble war in that they are frequently not directed against outgroups. They are not only regressive and cathartic but often intra-species responses.

Freud's description of the sources of group behavior have helped considerably in our understanding of the group. But he does not apply this illumination to the issue of the group behavior in war. Moreover one cannot accept his contention that war is the result of aggressive individual residues after civilization. This represents war as the product of the disorganization of the individual libido, a puerile symptom shared by many individuals. This is too simplistic a view, and neglects the group phenomena he elucidates.

On the contrary, war and other forms of organized violence, while they are rooted in primitive elemental forces, are firmly attached to the highest products of culture and civilization. It is with a particularly highly developed product that I am concerned which seems to me to be culpable of organized war. The product to which I refer is social identity. It provides the springs by which the cultured extra-group aggression is thrown up as organized phenomena.

The process of group acculturation includes as well the formation of individual and in-group identities, which provide the machinery for social action as well as for the culture of war. It is true however that certain problems or models of group identity are more likely than others to promote expression or to occasion group violence. The national form of group identity has proved to be a particularly dangerous and problematic model.

Among the chief potentials of the human being and among the chief goals of his acculturation is the production in him of his sense of identity, and the idea of self-in-the-group. I cannot here elaborate on the basic biological and on the complex cultural paths to social identity, mediated initially through negotiation with the figures in the family and other fostering groups.

Identity can become a catch-all concept but it does contain very pure elements of its own, this sense of the many-dimensional continuities of self and of belonging; of independence of the one and shared destiny and responsibility of the many. Identity develops as a balance between the esteem of self-in-the-group with the esteem of the self-by-the-group. Identity includes the sense of occupying physical and emotional space, binds itself to place and to time and impacts upon and reacts in particular ways with other similars and strangers. It is in its essence at the core of all personal and group existence and in its highest has been the preeminent human goal and content. It is, therefore, inescapably bound up with the crudest nature and the highest derivatives of human energy. In human identity, organic self-awareness is refined ultimately into the mirror complexities of human self and group esteem and evaluation.

It is to these qualities, those encapsulated in the concept of identity, to which one must appeal in order to understand the exhibition of organized human violence. Identity and esteem are inextricably both individual and group phenomena, just as is war. It is the group quality of identity which mobilizes the group culture for war.

My submission therefore is that war and organized violence are the inescapable product of the very highest reaches of our historic culture and the direct result of problems in or insults to the identity and self-esteem of the human group. War and organized group violence are more or less general reactions aimed at removing the source of threat to the identity and self-esteem of the group seeking violently to affirm or reaffirm group identity and self-esteem that threaten to fail. Violent responses may occur especially where the insult is brought to bear on an identity which is confused or hypertrophied. The insult is less likely, it appears, to elicit violence in identities which are securely lodged, unless survival is actually at stake.

It is the issue of identity and group culture rather than the purely hypnotic crowd response or an innate herd instinct which makes a cultured group of people ready for war and the tool of demagoguery or nationalist militarism. The acts of the culture of war are capable, however falsely, of reaffirming a failing group self-esteem and identity and of removing threats to it, real or phantasied. The floreat of a Hitler is not to be ascribed to a hypnotic dependence nor to primitive herd response nor yet to isolated libidinal or characterological fixations but to a total failure of the equilibria of self and group esteem of a total group.

Furthermore: It seems reasonable to assume that this postulation of problems in and insults to identity and self-esteem will help to explain many particular phenomena of violence and repeated violence, group or group-sanctioned, which have often been dismissed sophistically as *psychopathic* or *temperamental*. Vendettas and blood feuds are in this class. Clan and tribal warfare are too. The group violence of the culturally deprived and even the revolt of the Marxist Proletariat seeking to right an economic disadvantage do involve this element of identity, a class, economically deprived, finding a group identity.

Classes share identity with their (national) group. The generation of a new and over-riding group identity within a class, by virtue of its reaction to discrimination against it by another class, has much to add to the over-simplifications of dialectical history.

The problem for an emergent national group painfully making its way to a new identity is particularly sensitive. This is especially true of those national groups attempting to fuse a broader identity from preexisting tight kinship or ethnic identities. This process seems to be operating in the unrest and repetitive aggressive threats of the new Middle Eastern Arab States. On the other hand it seems that much of the general upheaval of values evident in the drug and sex revolt is a failed expression of an almost universal struggle of the new generations toward a new identity rising above that of the ingrown family, class and nation.

The vain struggles to establish an esteemed individual identity account a great deal for the decision to become an outlawed criminal or enter an outlawed criminal group. It certainly plays a great part in the process of becoming a prostitute in order to build up a new identity and to find a source of self-esteem. Addicts or alcoholics, in whom the violence is turned almost directly against the self, certainly seek their self-esteem and identity through drugs.

As has been submitted, human warfare and organized violence are to be lodged at the door of the modes of our group-based acculturation and of problems of identity and the failure of self-esteem. It seems therefore that we must look with real concern at the processes of identity of the individual in his family which are guided by the precepts of his national or near national group.

As has been so often felt, the national group is indeed an unsuitable crucible for the patterning of social values and of individual identity.

BIBLIOGRAPHY

1. Freud, S.: *Civilization and Its Discontents.* Hogarth, 1946, p. 90.
2. Freud: *op. cit.,* pp. 85-86, 102.
3. Lorenz, K.: *On Aggression.* Metheun, 1966, pp. 203-204.
4. Lorenz: *op. cit.,* p. 204.
5. Dollard, J. *et al.:* Kegan Paul, 1944, p. 1.
6. Freud, S.: *Group Psychology and the Analysis of the Ego.* Hogarth, 1940, pp. 1-20.

Chapter 14

PSYCHOANALYTIC OBSERVATIONS ON INTERNATIONAL CROSS-CURRENTS

ERIKA FREEMAN, Ed.D.

Introduction
John L. Carleton, M.D.

It is my guess that an aircraft manufacturing company approaches the construction of a new super-sonic plane by engaging a huge staff of specialized planning people who collect many, many facts and details which are then combined and utilized for the development of a master plan. Social psychiatry is embracing an area of involvement which is far vaster than airplane construction; yet we are only now beginning to identify and define specific parts of our area of involvement.

In our organization, the International Association for Social Psychiatry, we are attempting to accomplish some of this task. One of the great contributions of Erika Freeman is the vast number of ideas and concepts which flow from her most facile mind with such rapidity that one has to maintain extremely close attention or miss a great deal. Her discussion at the Santa Barbara Workshop, which is included here, is a typical example of this characteristic. Almost each and every sentence could become the theme of an ongoing research project which could provide important guidelines for government and society to follow for years to come. World survival is dependent upon this kind of information.

Let there be no mistake, social behavior scientists are in the forefront of the *now* revolution, the intellectual revolution, that is, and they are specifically involved in intellectual planning of goals and directions for society to follow. This may at first suggest authoritarian controls; however, on the contrary, greater freedom for each individual can only be assured if those responsible for the leadership and executive directions of government begin to devote greater and more careful attention to what is being said here and now.

In the early days of man, the demands of physical survival so limited his freedom that he could only think of better ways to avoid starvation and provide protection from the elements. All his energies, physical and mental, were necessarily devoted to these tasks. When the society grew prosperous enough to support teachers and thinkers, these people evolved and began to think about better ways of doing things, such as harnessing the energies of the universe. These to-be scientists have obviously made a great contribution. Perhaps simultaneously, there developed a group of thinkers and philosophers who were to become the behavioral scientists and physicians. Religion and psychology developed as an outgrowth and in response to the humanistic needs of all people. Religion is, of course, among other things, a way of providing guidelines and controlling basic human instinctual behavior. Religion can be compared to a kind of psychotherapy except that its insights have, in the past, been limited. The modern psychotherapist does not employ magic, and his rituals are hopefully designed only to facilitate more authentic insights rather than simply strengthen repression or repressive ego defenses. These de-repressive methods open up progressively new worlds for people to explore. Thus, it is fair to say that Erika's paper is offering directions which can lead to these insights, at not only an individual but also at an international level. National governments and other organizations, we emphasize, must pay attention and support further exploration of these insights.

THE INTERESTING THING about international tensions is that they start with national tensions which in turn start with intranational tensions which are intrapersonal tensions. The tensions which we have with each other are easily noticed because they have to do with our own psyche, with the way we perceive the world. It is less easy to see, however, that in all international conflict intrapsychic mechanisms are at work.

You will have to forgive my psychoanalytic bias and excuse my use of a number of words in a way which may seem to be jargonese. I might utilize my use of language as one example of all the things, in this case, language, which contribute to interpersonal tensions and international tensions. Language can be used in several ways, in the case of English, as common English or as the specialist's *jargon*. Hence, when we are thinking of international cross-currents we are dealing with differences between languages as well as differences of language usage within one given language. Thus we are at a double loss.

Another major difficulty we face in international understanding concerns the information we get from other countries. The case is similar as with languages. It is difficult to gain information about disciplines other than one's own even within one's country.

But for what goes on with professionals outside, in other countries, we rely on newspapers, periodicals or bibliographies, and therefore we rely on what newsmen or bibliographers think is worth publishing, translating, or printing. Moreover, what we are not conditioned to hear about other countries we refuse to believe, partly because of our own prejudices and biases, partly because of our interests and leanings. For we do have a tendency to pay greater attention to those things for which we have an affinity.

This includes the images which we have of certain countries. Let me give you an example of one judgment by *image*. Last week the *New York Times* had an article about four-year-old children learning to play in a nursery school. For fifteen or twenty minutes twice a day the children did calisthenics in the schoolyard, each child learning to handle a little wooden rifle. The author of this article was quite friendly to this kind of schooling. I am deliberately telling you this story backwards to let your prejudices work on it. You see, the author was a Swede, and the country about whose children he wrote was Red China. For when you hear of children being trained in using guns, you don't think of Red China, the mystical god of the New Revolution. Likewise, you don't expect a Swedish anthropologist to approve of war, after all, Sweden is giving refuge to our youth who do not wish to be involved in the Vietnam War.

What is so sad about this, and it happens in all countries, is that we take ideas from countries we like and do not accept notions and commitments of or even compromises with countries we do not like. Indeed, we go so far as to accept terrible ideas, bad policy, from countries we like. In terms of our national as well as international relations, such guidance by inclinations has disastrous results. Ultimately, of course, I could reduce such international policy as determined by inclination or personal idiosyncracy down to saying that Nixon's America is not Kennedy's, De Gaul's France is not Pompidou's.

To summarize: we don't care about the content of policy, of what is good or bad, but rather about who represents the policy. Thus we get into wars for causes, notions and personalities which actually are personal causes, or inclinations of our politicians, but which may be totally alien to us as a nation—a fact which explains why we have alliances with an odd assortment of nations.

In American politics you might also trace the development of personal political idiosyncrasies to a man's family background. A second generation American may dislike and distrust his father's country of origin, or he may cherish his relationship to his father and his father's to his country.

We are more interested in, more drawn to those political notions and actions which are most closely allied to our own psychological structure. All these matters make the problem of international relations incredibly complex. Moreover, in some respects our psychological structure includes a certain kind of morbidity or pathology. One of the dangers we must combat is putting our pathology in the service of politics. For instance, it is a rationalization to say, "Well, we're blowing you up for your own good. If you die, it'll be better for you because ultimately it's better to be dead than red."

Aside from being a meaningless slogan, "better dead than red" says that it is better to be dead than anything that does not agree with my temporary ideas. I had hopes that, by this time, we would no longer say this. But we do. We still are drawn to ideas which appeal to our psyches. More importantly, we are drawn to countries with whom we are told to be friendly. And, by paradox, we are also drawn to countries who are our declared enemies. We pay more attention to what the Russians or the Chinese are doing, or to what we think they are doing, or to what we are predisposed to wish they are doing than to what the African nations are doing. I deliberately point to the major powers because they are the large enemy and we have a kind of symbiotic relationship with them. We seem to depend on each other for our opinions. If the Russians think one thing, we think another. In fact, we are more concerned with what they are doing than with what we are doing. We are more concerned with what another country of our size does than we are concerned with Colombia, Peru or Mexico or indeed our former enemies, Germany and Japan.

And built into these notions and everybody else's notions, into the personal longings and the needs of the personal psyche is another factor, the factor of cultural disposition. I am thinking of something much like Erikson's suggestion that each culture creates personalities which are viable within that culture, structured to survive in that culture.

We as psychoanalysts and as mental health workers do not believe that adjustment *per se* is a good thing if the adjustment is to pathology (whether it be personal or cultural pathology). We also believe that a free choice is good. (By free I mean an educated and reasonable choice in human relations and activities.) We want to give individuals and, ultimately, nations a choice. We want to free them from being driven by their unconscious pathologies. Some people seem to insist that historical necessity operates in the relationships of nations to one another. I suggest that this historical necessity ultimately is due to personal pathology. If everybody had tuberculosis and if everybody adjusted to tuberculosis, everybody would be ill and not healthy.

For instance, two people are determined to get something but they have opposing political ideas, let us say Hitler and a social democrat opponent of his in 1933. Unfortunately the latter's immediate energy for acting upon his ideas is not as great as the pathological energy available to Hitler by reason of his obsession and compulsivity. If one questions how can a man like Hitler come to be head of state the answer is simple: his energy was greater; he was more perservering, more intense and incidentally, more pathological. And unfortunately pathology is contagious but sanity and health could be contagious as well. In a sense we don't teach health because we don't call attention to it; we take it for granted. We point to a man's acting irrationally, idiotically. The more we call attention to it, the more we are teaching about it. It does not seem a reasonable alternative to teach about the man who sits and works in a university, a court house or a hospital. That is too simple, and none of us are so original as to broadcast that as an alternative.

We only know those alternatives that we are taught, that we hear about, read about, speak about. When we suggest that violence in this country is an alternative we already teach that it *is* an alternative. But some alternatives are not really alternatives.

I have not heard anyone saying that violence is not an alternative —it is a resort to pathological behavior. It is not a viable alternative. It is something you do—it comes up in negotiations. We have come to assume in our country that one of the ways in which you negotiate is to say either you do this or there will be violence. We don't say "you either take three steps or you take five steps." We say "you either take three steps or violence." We do not teach that violence is not an alternative, that the either/ or is not appropriate, and by such neglect we ignore our responsibility.

I know it has become extremely fashionable to hold certain notions and more than that to express these notions in a particular way, for instance either/or is *in*, and must be expressed violently; or the word *revolutionary* is good; anyone else is bad as in Orwell's animal farm, "two legs bad, four legs good." Moreover, if you don't use revolutionary jargon (even if you share some of the *revolutionary* conclusions), you are not *one of us*, or if you have arrived at some similar conclusions as the *revolutionaries* but by different roads, your own roads, you are not *my fellow*. You don't belong to the *revolutionary* movement of today if you don't use four-letter words, do not use violence, do not say that automatically black is good, white is trash. There is something in the insistence upon blackness, whiteness, Japaneseness, *revolutionariness* which violates the principle of human equality—for this insistence forces us into uniformity while it claims to resolve our differences. Possibly the way in which people are equal is the way in which they have a right to be different, different from each other, different within themselves.

Why the intolerence, why the either this or violence? Now one of the difficulties we as psychoanalysts have, a difficulty which does not exist for classical physics or for the man of common sense, is the problem of paradox. For them it is simple: two opposing matters or situations or facts cannot exist in the same place at the same time. We know exactly the opposite: two opposing feelings about the same subject can and do exist in the same person at the same time. We call it ambivalence and we have to live with it. Most adults learn to live with ambivalence but when they get frightened they seem to need the either/or alternatives.

That is to say, under stress many people tend to regress and for the child in us the either/or alternative is more comfortable. For to children we explain matters by saying that they are either this or that, knowing that for the mature person matters are, all things being equal, neither this nor that but rather some of this and some of that. This is a tacit assumption for us but as Margaret Mead says: "everybody knows, but nobody says; nobody says, nobody knows." Thus what *we* take for granted, other people will not take for granted and will insist on their either/or alternatives.

Similarly, the next generation will not take for granted our experience and the reasons for our conclusions. All they have are the conclusions themselves. On these they base their future. Youth is not interested in the past, in the way we reached our conclusions. Part of being young is to have the kind of energy that says "never mind yesterday, what about tomorrow." Well, our problems are today and I suppose the best cure for today is tomorrow—providing there is a tomorrow.

But what influences tomorrow's goals? What tomorrows do we choose and why? Let me suggest that a country's vision of its tomorrow (and different countries' visions of their tomorrows are fortunately not that different) depends on its relationship to another countries' vision of its tomorrow. Basically I posit that countries are to each other what humans are to each other; they are family constellations. For instance, once upon a time, England was the mother country of the world; today she is a grandmother. Once she had a powerful role but now, although she lacks the power she still knows it all, has all the advice, is not yet senile.

Then we have parent countries, but these are continually changing. At present Russia and America are the parent countries. The difficulty of the United States in being a parent country is that it is still an adolescent if you consider its psychological structure. In terms of adolescence, it is what Goethe used to call: "Himmelhoch jauchzend, zu Tode betrübt"—or sky-high with happiness, depressed unto death. Aside from being a hallmark of adolescence this mood is also indicative of creativity. I suppose in order to remain creative one has to remain reasonably unsettled and be unsettled within reason, willing to grow and to continue searching, yet without finding the search so fearful that one becomes afraid and falls for any slogan that promises a total solution or a total answer to one's search.

Now, I believe we have to watch out when we are looking for answers from other people or other peoples. Fortunately, most of us here are international. That is to say, one of the unique things in this country is that we all came from different national backgrounds and hence, in listening to answers, most likely we do not hear the same things. This fact makes for a more varied capacity for absorption of different ideas from different countries. Nevertheless, we have to watch out for our unconscious biases and, in relating to each other and to other countries, agree upon a rational sequence that we can mutually understand and according to which we can anticipate each other's actions. We should remember that we tend to have an opinion or to take action before we have really understood the other person's viewpoint and have made a rational assessment of the situation.

Let us take as an example the young revolutionary of today—or the so-called revolutionary. He says *not later—now* with an impatience that we associate with infantilism. Not that things do not need doing immediately but if you ask, "Oh, not later, now; but what?" and the answer is "I don't know, but not what you are doing," then you know that you are not speaking to a revolutionary. Really revolutionary ideas are these: we are not in control, we do not really know what is going on, we are entitled to search for new answers; things are not acceptable as they are and we don't have any pat answer. Submission to slogans will not help us.

Revolution in this country as I see it does not concern that which we are supposed to abhor such as violence, bloodshed, killing of victim people X rather than Y. Revolution is concerned with changing to better ways of living, of thinking, of relating to others. Revolution demands of us a total concern for the individual.

Hence the term revolutionary does not designate anything as *irrelevant,* a word which has become prevalent and which is applied to whatever anyone wishes. I suggest that the notion of irrelevance is one of the great dangers to the human psyche, to the human personality, to personal freedom. What is human or concerns humans cannot be irrelevant for there are no experts on the future. Since creative solutions, by definition, have got to be radically new and different, they cannot be legislated in advance or labelled by slogans such as *irrelevant* in advance. Suppose a legislator had come to James Watt and said, "why are you fiddling around with all that steam, what is it good for?" The creative solution is such a leap that it is alien, perhaps frivolous, to what is now, but we need it for tomorrow.

In terms of the U.S. as a parent country with an adolescent psychic structure our problems are many more than I outlined. Let me add another few.* Yesterday we talked about the nature of political—or psychological—communication or the lack of it by the use of obscenity. (We call communication political if it is from country to country, psychological if it is from person to person.) Note that in our culture obscenity is equated with sexual behavior and not, for instance, with sitting in Siberia or with the genocide of the Watusi.

Now, obscenity, if you don't get frightened by its sexual implications, is a useful and very effective way of getting attention and therefore of eventually communicating. If the young people are using obscenity it is because they have been trying to talk to their parents, their teachers, anybody, but nobody has paid any attention. Have young people use an expletive and suddenly the entire older generation listens! "Hey, guess what! They paid attention."

Now, if we pay attention only when youth talk to us by obscenity we have taught them to relate to us in that manner. If we refuse to listen to reason, logic, sense, we are teaching youth to be unreasonable, illogical, offensive. For young people this kind of attention is unrewarding; it is negative attention. The adult who came to listen to the obscene prelude thinks: "Well, if he talks like that I am not going to listen to him." You cannot blame the young person for using that type of prelude. Besides, he cannot be sure that he will not get through.

Let me give you another communication problem. Intellectually all of us here in this room agree that all men are created equal and are entitled to the same rights and privileges. We be-

* See Professor Harry Girvetz's paper, "Anatomy of Violence."

lieve we are reasonable, helpful and useful, saviors of the world. Yesterday, however, we all showed how thin that veneer is when it looked as if two speakers, metaphorically speaking, might draw blood. I would have been fascinated to see how a man of Dr. Brill's experience utilizes a confrontation and converts the hostility generated and uses it constructively.

Instead, the emotional drive of our meeting was "no, don't interrupt, Dr. Brill, let them get at it." We acted as if we were going to be deprived of a major spectacle. In a sense, we gave in to that irrational part in us which really does not want to solve problems, which really wants to convert anyone into an enemy and refuses to have this enemy taken away from him. Hence our irrationality for a time led us to assume the wrong kind of enemies. We have to posit the right kinds of enemies because, heaven knows, we have enough enemies. What then are our right enemies? Poverty and ignorance.

In fact, ignorance these days is a double problem as it has come to be respected. Note the following example: someone comes to my husband's studio and says "I don't know anything about art but I know what I like." What this man really says is: respect my ignorance and pay it the same homage as you expect me to pay to your education in art. We need to face the problem that ignorance can become a vice for it keeps us narrow, hence frightened. The more frightened we become, the more violent we become; the more enemies we make, the less we are able to do for others.

Some of our intellectuals seem to be ashamed of the discipline it took to become more human and they say that it is ignorance we should be after. Yet once you have learned something you cannot become ignorant again; once you know something you carry responsibility. That is why you might be attracted by ignorance, for it promises freedom from responsibility.

To come back to my early hypothesis concerning parent-countries. Being a country with mothering functions means to have greater responsibility and being less able to afford ignorance. Being a parent country may mean for some people having greater rank and privilege than other countries. It may also mean being accused of wanting to run the world. But neither need be the motive for behavior as a parent country, for feeling responsible for the world. We need to keep in mind that, as parents, countries will take their turn and will abdicate the parent's role when they are no longer needed. Hence, we can all be each other's teachers and learn from each other. Thus we might learn from England's successes as well as her failures as a parent country, and she was a more stable parent than most.

I also believe that, in the long run, a democratic country makes a better parent than a fascist country. In a fascist country rules are external, they are clear. You may do this, you may not do this —or else. In a democratic country rules are not clear cut but flexible, decided on in particular cases by mutual agreement. Living by such rules requires some self-discipline, some judgment, patience, flexibility, insight into the options available. If a democratic parent country can instill into younger countries such attitudes these countries will in any case be stabler and less violent. If a democratic country feels entitled to be autocratic with younger countries (since *they* have not yet arrived at a stage where democracy comes easily), the parent country is making a bad mistake.

Let me summarize: In making political judgments we should be aware of the complexity of personal and interpersonal psychological factors that influence political behavior, whether national or international. The developmental stage of persons or countries who influence or make political decisions vitally contributes to the political process. Last but not least, the traits of the individual who copes with the world knowledgeably and realistically are the same traits that enable countries to live in a community of nations.

Chapter 15

THE DRAFT AND COMMUNITY MENTAL HEALTH

J. B. TIETZ, LL.B.

MY CONTRIBUTION this morning is to present for your consideration observations and opinions based on my experiences. I presume I have been chosen to participate in this workshop because my work has long been in a unique specialty where many men, and their families, are enduring emotional stresses that should, and can, be mitigated.

My daily work is to aid men who do not wish to enter military service and to aid men who want out of the armed forces.

It is a fact of current American life that the men I deal with and their families represent a significant portion of our population. We are only tangentially concerned with their reasons for refusal of military service.

This paper presents opinions and factual matter to aid you in understanding how the mental health of two closely related classes of young men and their families can be improved.

My work for most of the last twenty-seven years, and for all of the last six, has dealt with draft age men who have a deferment problem with the Selective Service System chiefly because they have conscientious objections to serving their country in its armed organizations. I also assist a second class of young men, who are in an even more trying situation, as their problem is with one of the armed services, which they have joined either by enlistment or induction. The problem facing each of the men in this second class is that his conscience has developed, finally matured, ripened, crystallized, and become fixed after his entry into the armed service, and it no longer permits him to remain there.

Since both classes of these young men, and their loved ones, total at the very least many tens of thousands, their problems deserve the attention of this assemblage. Not to be overlooked, are the many additional tens of thousands of concerned persons, who, although having no relatives directly involved, are yet greatly disturbed by the predicaments of these people. These latter persons are like the abolitionists of 150 years ago who declared "I am not free when others are enslaved." Their anguish and emotional disturbance is real.

In short, all the young men, their relatives and their sympathizers have emotional problems that range from anxiety to neurosis to psychosis.

To restate, and sharpen our focus, I will deal here today as I do seven days a week with two groups: those who do not wish to be drafted, chiefly by reason of conscientious objection; and those already in the armed services who want out, chiefly by reason of conscientious objection.

I now examine the problem of each of the two classes of young men and thereafter proceed to suggest remedies.

The Problems

First, the Draft

The government has always recognized that problems of very considerable size exist with the draft, and today, more than ever, it is doing something about it.[1] I shall take a few minutes on this and then express my view, namely, that not enough is being done.

At all times during this century our draft laws have provided for deferments and exemptions which in our time have given a measure of relief from anxiety to a total of 20,000,000[2] men and their families. Briefly, out of 40,000,000 registrants since 1948 many millions were out of draft danger long before the induction date. Over 5,000,000 did not meet the medical and other military standards of acceptability. Many millions more fairly quickly secured deferments such as III-A, meaning that their induction would bring extreme hardship to their families. The list of deferments has been lengthy, and includes those in my principal field of work, the 40,000 conscientious objectors.

Second, the Military

Also, at all times during this century, military regulations have provided for release of both enlistees and inductees in hardship and other categories[3] and, in the last nine years, for men who become conscientious objectors after entering the armed services.[4]

Since considerable avenues of relief are open, and relief has already been attained by many, what is the size of the present problem and what is the government doing about it? Also, what are others doing about what the government cannot do because of its responsibilities for national defense?

After watching these matters closely for over twenty-seven years, I am satisfied that more opposition to entering the armed services exists today than ever before, that a comparable ratio of drafted men who are in the armed services are like-minded, and that a considerable number of volunteers, especially ROTC and other junior commissioned officers, also have come to the position that they can no longer stay in military life. The facts are quite well known; this belief is shared by very many and I presume that is why I was invited to speak here. I take it then that all here have at least an academic interest in this matter and/or professional concern, or an experiential involvement, personal or family.

We all know that many antimilitary sentiments are widespread among great numbers of young men (Senator McGovern on February 28, 1971, expressed the opinion on television that the majority of Americans share them). In any event, here are some comments we hear from young men:

How will my family fare while I'm away? or

How can I take part in this war, one I consider oppressive, unjust and a national calamity? or

How can I take part in any war, an activity I consider contrary to the dictates of my conscience?

We are also sadly aware of certain solutions chosen, namely, that thousands of our young men have gone into exile (likely permanent) to Canada;[5] a considerable number have chosen an *underground* life, continually hiding from recognition; and worse yet, the suicide rate of males aged eighteen to twenty-six has risen sharply in the past five years.[6]

The list is longer than the types I mention, but the half dozen items I refer to above present enough to give an indication of the population affected both quantitatively and qualitatively. It is true that many governmental agencies are intensifying their efforts to meet this problem, and after a headline-type review I'll proceed with what is yet needed, and why.

We are aware that the Navy has been radically modernizing its attitudes to its personnel,[7] although the Army is making less energetic efforts in the same direction;[8] that the Marine Corps claims some progress; and that the Selective Service System is telling the world it is giving itself a new look.[9] Of course, the only thing that could completely allay the particular anxieties we deal with this morning is a total renunciation of the draft and a state of world-wide peace.

Although many are working for those goals, we here are required to consider and should only consider today the avoidable tension problems caused by the draft and the armed forces.

First, I deal with the draft. Everyone here probably knows that statistically the chances of being drafted until a year ago were fifty-fifty; this percentage is due alone to deferments and to the physical and mental acceptability standards. We also know that the odds have changed considerably by reason of the lottery. By the lottery alone the odds changed to twenty-five/seventy-five, one chance in four; and by reason of other factors it is today even a trifle better.

But, as we all know, while on the one hand youth, and even people generally, tend to think that ill luck is what befalls others, on the other hand many registrants and their families are always concerned with the draft, a substantial number for very good reasons. The good reasons are (1) that they have been found acceptable by the military doctors at the preinduction physical examination, (2) that their lottery numbers are under 196; (3) that by reason of unpredictable international climate their period of draft exposure can be extended; and (4) that many consider the draft lottery as unfair as a lottery on income tax would be.

I shall first detail the more important current efforts made to reduce the tensions of the draft system on the civilian population and later, the current efforts of the military.

Many changes were instituted during the last three years to minimize dissatisfaction with the draft and its methods of operation. Some changes not only did not minimize dissatisfaction but increased it. Let me give two quick examples. When the President, in the exercise of the power delegated to him in the Act of Congress, eliminated occupational and some other deferments on April 23, 1970, his added statement that he desired Congress to give back to him the delegated power he once had to eliminate student deferments, this threat, this actual prospect, now facing *all* high school graduates was disturbing to many families; second, with respect to the April 23rd elimination of new occupational deferments, many more persons were alarmed. The Scientific Manpower Commission eventually expressed its great concern that there would soon be a crippling shortage of trained engineers.[10] Dr. Tarr's answer was that the President *might*, in the future, authorize occupational deferments.[11]

It can be concluded that the only *successful* change was the lottery. Eventually, after stumbling for months, it gave a large portion of the affected population peace of mind.

This was a good step for the lucky ones, but what of the remainder, the low number men? They with their families total many hundred thousands.

So, what is being done? Let me canvass the three governmental branches:

The executive branch through its administrative agency, the SSS, has recently been working towards a better public image which, if resolutely implemented, would have the effect of relieving some of the tensions that bring about today's mental health concern. I will detail this soon.

The judicial branch has only an incidental impact; its part is too specialized to be catalogued in this paper other than to say that many of its decisions, such as *Welsh*,[12] have given new hope to a considerable number of people.

The legislative branch has done nothing final. It will be compelled to legislate on the subject because the military concedes it cannot get along without the draft for at least a year or two. The time, therefore, is here when you, as individuals, and as influential members of learned societies, can form opinions and then express to the legislature, both your Senators and your Congressmen, your special concerns.

The administrative agency, the Selective Service System, is currently engaged in a public relations program unprecedented in its history. Its program includes the announcement that it is welcoming suggestions from all; it already is mailing a very large array of informational material for registrants and their parents, to high school principals and to draft counselors in schools, colleges and unattached private counseling centers and counselors.

A unique part of its effort is the explicit and direct wooing of the counseling groups that oppose the draft and particularly the old, large, prestigious pacifist organizations. Some of these national religious or pacifist organizations have always had good working relations with the System's national office and with the Pentagon and with the Department of Justice. It is new, however, to have the System affirmatively attempt to enlist cooperation of these national bodies and, even more surprising, to also attempt to enlist the cooperation of the myriad of small, autonomous and unaffiliated local counseling bodies. Additionally, the printed material now possessed by the System is being sent out to anyone who requests it.

What we should consider is: are these and similar efforts to create a better image likely to ameliorate tensions, or not? If not, what can we do?

These efforts of the director have been viewed with suspicion. This reaction is reported in the periodicals and news letters of the large, experienced groups. Some of the smaller groups jeer and lampoon, as before. What the outcome will be cannot confidently be predicted at this moment. There is sufficient evidence on hand to believe that the cooperation of *none* of the pacifist and other *anti-draft* organizations will be gained. For one thing, doubt of sincerity is being expressed. It is clear, the concerned pacifists say, that the present public policy of the System is solely to improve its image, to make the System more palatable.

It must be kept in mind that Dr. Tarr is an advocate; he is like a lawyer who knows, must know, only his client. He is not a judge; he certainly is no longer a professor, and, like this member of your panel, can make no pretense of ivory tower detachment from the fray.

I will summarize by selected sentences what each of the two oldest and most active pacifist organizations has to say before presenting the evidence on which I base my conclusions.

A. The Central Committee for Conscientious Objectors Newsletter[13] says:

> After nearly three decades of a Selective Service System under General Hershey that did its best to keep men from learning their options and rights, it is hard not to praise any serious effort by Selective Service to explain the draft in simple language, in enough detail to let men plan their lives with some awareness of their choices, and with recognition of the nonmilitary as well as the military alternatives.
>
> Second, the booklets omit huge amounts of essential information and don't suggest any other sources. . . .
>
> Third, all the booklets have serious inaccuracies, as well as many of the minor errors that tell you they were prepared by new, inexperienced employees. . . .

B. The National Interreligious Service Board for Conscientious Objectors also expresses serious doubts concerning the objectivity and even-handedness of the System's new look.[14] I quote three sentences:

> In testimony before the [house sub-] committee, the draft chief complained that many counselors and lawyers were aiding registrants to escape the draft "by emphasizing in the courts the nonlegal nature with which we do our work." Attorneys and counselors are mentioned by name in the testimony as advertising that they "can assure a client for a fee that he will be able to avoid a legal obligation." Nearly fifteen pages of the report is taken up with transcripts of speeches and newspaper articles by these attorneys and counselors. . . .
>
> Said Dr. Tarr, "The spread of draft counseling is certainly one of the most alarming changes in America as it relates to the draft right now."
>
> Tarr's testimony appears to run strikingly counter to recent public announcements from Selective Service National Office which invite counselors to "join forces to insure that all young men are provided with complete, straightforward information on the draft."

The unmistakable conclusion is that Dr. Tarr cannot count on the assistance of any of the pacifist organizations in what should be an effort to allay suspicion and fear.

In addition to opinions of the above pacifist organizations there is other evidence for belief that Dr. Tarr is concerned one hundred percent with the fundamental aims of the System, and not visibly with the mental health concerns of the group assembled here today.

First, he instinctively takes a hard line. Immediately after the Supreme Court decided *Welsh,* by that decision eliminating the necessity of a religious basis for conscientious objection, he took to the air and said, of such a registrant: "His belief must be the result of some kind of rigorous training." This statement was repeated on the front pages of newspapers the next two days, in quotation marks.

This statement, whether thoughtfully intended or not, certainly gave the boards an easy out. They could now make a finding, after consideration of an applicant's evidence, that he had training but that it wasn't *rigorous* enough. This is similar, although not legally parallel, to the tightening-up change made in the regulations in 1951 from *hardship* to *extreme hardship,* for the III-A classification.

Evidently Dr. Tarr's legal advisors immediately were alarmed and must have informed him that there was no statutory basis for inclusion of the expression *rigorous.* Therefore, when the regulation came out in print his imported, artificial, arbitrary and illegal standard was not present.

I assert he had already planted a seed in the receptive memories of the board members. I am satisfied that it is now understood by the board members that, by the use of the one word *insincere,* they can defeat the conscientious objection applicant. This is already happening in the trials of these cases.

I concede that perhaps a man should not forever be held accountable for just one remark. So, let us examine his subsequent conduct.

Next, the director appeared on a TV program on November 24, 1970, and said, "The difficulty on conscientious objection is always determining who is sincere, who is actually making a profession on the basis of his conscience. This difficulty is one that jurors and judges face every day. It is no argument against the jury system."

Next, consider his testimony at the Hearings of the Special
Subcommittee on the Draft of the Committee on Armed Services.
Congressman Hebert of Louisiana was chairman until recently,
when he became head of the main committee, that is, the Committee on Armed Forces, due to the death of Mendel Rivers.

To evaluate what I will soon be quoting it is essential to keep
in mind the new look the director has been giving the System by
wooing the pacifist and other groups opposing the draft. This
I described above. While he was wooing, he testified to the subcommittee as reported on page 12,471 of the proceedings that
ended November 18, 1970:

> The campaign of disruption goes on, and in terms of physical costs
> alone it is expensive. In many cities and towns draft counseling
> services have been set up to encourage registrants to use various
> delaying actions in classification processes. *In Oakland, California,
> just a week ago, I was alarmed to see the draft counseling offices
> across the street from our large Armed Forces Examining and En-
> trance Station.*

From the above you can see why I look at Dr. Tarr as I do a
United States Attorney; he is an advocate. He has his job to do
and no one can look to him to lessen tensions unless it incidentally
aids his principal purpose.

While life presents many bases for anxieties to all of us, the
young men of today, and their families, have special twin anxieties,
the draft and the military.

I will not attempt to catalog and discuss the components; the
time allotted this paper is too short. I will take what I consider the
chief one in each of these two areas, military and draft, and deal
with each item in some detail.

Now, the military. It is usually known to every enlistee and
every inductee who wants out of the military that the law provides several avenues of release, such as extreme hardship to
close relatives, various kinds of unsuitability, and conscientious
objection.[15] It is also known that each application faces an obstacle course. It could not be otherwise. I will deal only with the
attainable.

This morning I deal with only one of the bases for relief,
namely conscientious objection. Before I get to my precise point

we should all be familiar with some of the history of release by reason of conscientious objection.

In 1962 the Department of Defense issued a directive providing "for the honorable discharge of personnel who became conscientious objectors." This is DoD 1300.6. It required all the armed services, the four regular ones and the seven reserve and guard outfits, to implement the directive by its own regulations. All eleven are substantially alike and follow the wording of the DoD.

For three or four years this policy worked reasonably well but as Vietnam escalated the policy was sabotaged at the local level, perhaps everywhere. This sabotage and the resulting outcry produced an amendment to the DoD in 1968 that considerably ameliorated the situation. The chief items of change were that the initial interview was transferred from the applicant's commanding officer to *a knowledgeable officer 03 or higher* and that the applicant could be represented by private counsel. While it took a good many months for the printed regulations to reach grass roots, and many installations either had no *knowledgeable* captain or officer of higher rank the duty eventually was given to a legal officer. Many of them soon became expert at this work.

All during the past several years, each time I visited Fort Ord for a 03 hearing or for a courtmartial, I inquired of all I met about the conscientious objector population. Always I was told, "There are about two hundred of us here."

With this background I will now point out one of the most important reasons why conscientious objection has become a considerable problem to the army and of concern and even anguish to many people.

At all times, in the last quarter century, comments like the following have appeared in the letters or other written statements given me. The one I now quote appears in a client's AR 635-20 application for c.o. discharge:

> During basic training, we spent most of our time just worrying about how we could keep out of trouble. It seemed that everything you did was wrong. We had little time to think about if what we were doing was right because they kept us constantly busy and very tired. . . .
>
> In bayonet training they made us say "Kill, Kill, Kill" as loud as

we could but it sounded so sadistic I just said "Hill, Hill, Hill" to
sort of make a game of it. It was a joke to me until I figured out
they really meant it. So "Hill" was what I said because I knew I
would never kill—so why even start acting like it. I convinced a
few of my close friends to say "Hill" too.

There are two elements of this particular subject that we
should consider: is such brutalizing necessary and is it worth it?

They can be considered together. Take the familiar fact of the
soldier named Meadlo, the young man who recently testified,
after having been given immunity, that he and Lt. Calley shot
down over one hundred women and children at My Lai. We
should recall the comment of Meadlo's mother, reported in the
newspapers: "I sent them a good boy; they sent me back a mur-
derer."

We have the recent report in the Scientific Manpower Commission's January, 1971, publication called *Manpower Comments,*
Vol. 8, No. 1, at page 23:

> Dr. Charles J. Leavy, Harvard research psychiatrist who spent two
> years working with returning Vietnam veterans, testified before the
> Senate Veteran Affairs Subcommittee that a *"boot camp in reverse"*
> *should be created to make returning combat troops less violent be-*
> *fore they reenter civilian life.* Leavy said that men returning from
> Vietnam suffer profound disorientation in some cases, and some
> were unable to distinguish between Vietnam and the community
> to which they returned.

It needs no further discussion that military training presents
an emotional problem to many of the men and to their families.

Is such brutalizing really necessary? I have long held the belief that bayonet training is given too soon to recruits and is too
frequently conducted by men who should not be given this work.

The Marine Corps, for example, has historically prided itself
on the slogan *every man a fighter.* It is well known to all newspaper readers that the Corps has had repetitious incidents of
trouble with unnecessarily brutal sergeants; also, that its desertion
rate is far higher than any of the other armed services. These matters are frequently the subject of press items. Is all this to its
credit? Are these methods necessary for the development of an
assault body? This is doubtful for, at least publicly, the Corps
has seen a need to maintain a *good* public image by the

announced transfer or court martial of the drill sergeant who has become the subject of a newspaper story. Also, the experience of the Israeli armed forces is that brutality and ridiculous shouting during bayonet training is unnecessary.[16]

These matters seem to be among the subjects of current inquiry by the armed services and considerable changes in military life and discipline are said to be under way.

Conclusions

The following remedial suggestions are not intended to be definitive and a panacea.

The Draft Law

It should be abolished. If not, sweeping reforms are required:

a. The determination of certain classification entitlements, such as for Class I-O (conscientious objection) should be delegated to independent and more expert bodies, such as the system used by England, when it had conscription[17] and such as presently used by the Selective Service System for the determination of Class I-Y (medically, morally or intellectually unsuitable registrants) namely the AFEES installations.[18]

b. Meetings with the boards: (1) An appealing registrant should have the right to appear before the Appeal Board. (2) A hearing before a local board should include the right to have witnesses and to have a lawyer's assistance. (3) The boards, local and appeal, must give an explicit reason, factually supported, for an adverse decision.

c. Except in time of declared wars all hardship deferments should be available.

d. There should be a nationwide trial of the following plan: men who file conscientious objector claims should automatically be assigned to one of the several ecological or reconstruction organizations, similar to VISTA, etc.

e. Attention must be given to the fact that a shockingly high percentage of our men, 19 to 26 years old, are rejected by reason of army standards, almost all medical. AR 40-501 [see footnote 2].

Sending these men out of the AFEES (examining station) whether happy or dejected is wrong: there should be (1) some advice and (2) a mandatory, periodic checkup with a written report required from the young man on his corrective effort. This can then be transferred to the Department of H.E.W. for analysis with [general] remedial and preventive recommendations to Congress.

f. *National* service should be further considered. Women are essential to the national welfare. If there is validity to the reason given for the proposal of health followup, made immediately above, attention to women-power is a corollary.

g. Draft Counseling Centers: They should be supervised much as are medical centers and high schools (for accreditation). Too many are staffed by the semi-ignorant.[19] They exist because there is an unquenched thirst, a genuine need, for information; and, until recently the SSS has done nothing about it. Even at present, with its surprising effort to make great quantities of factual material available, it is still suspect in many quarters.

How to remedy this: ombudsman-like area Consultation Clearance Boards, each with one stenographer, can be used and their *imprimatur* would provide better guidance. These boards could be composed of one SSS official (preferably a Supervising Executive Secretary, on a rotating basis) and one executive from each of the following groups: labor, employers, an old line pacifist organization, and a lawyer recommended by the local federal judges [the federal courts alone handle draft cases]. Such men and women are available in all principal sections of the country and would serve, unpaid, as draft board members do.

Military Reform

a. The well-published *proposed* changes should be implemented by a congressional mandate. The Colonel Blimps that abound must have brought home to them that civilian law attitudes, not ignorant and arbitrary decisions, are to be the rule. For example, the legal officers should be consulted (and, where possible, used) in all cases involving a legal problem. Illustrative instances: in Vietnam private counsel have been unnecessarily hindered in meeting and consulting with clients.[20] In in-service hearings for conscientious objector discharge at many of the military installations *line* officers, believing they can understand the regulations, have forbidden taping of the hearings, furnishing counsel with a copy of their recommendations, etc. Legal officers understand the court's interpretations and do not make such blatant and unnecessary errors which result in unnecessary litigation and end in court reversals of such improper military conduct.[21]

b. These in-service hearings should be speeded up so that the applicant need not be kept in limbo for the many months now taken. This is especially true of guard and reservist organizations.

There should be a direct order that provides for a time schedule for each step so that the unit confronted with such a request, novel to it, does not shelve it until polite threats of bringing the Inspector General into the picture get action.

A time schedule is necessary and one or more reviewing steps can be eliminated in that they are made solely on a paper record and too frequently result merely in a *pro forma* rejection, one without a rime or reason given.

c. Every hearing officer should be a *qualified* man just as the defense counsel in a serious court martial must be a lawyer.

The regulations of each service *require* that the 03 Hearing Officer be *knowledgeable*. Most of the unnecessary difficulties that have arisen are due to the word *knowledgeable*. Breathes there an officer with ego so dead that he doesn't believe he can understand English?

In the larger military installations there is a legal office, Judge Advocate General. JAG men can readily become knowledgeable for they know [item one] that the meanings of all regulations have likely been construed by the courts and [item two] that what the courts say is the meaning that governs, until such time when [item three] the law and/or regulations promulgated under the law's direction are amended. The line officer seems to have no conception of these three items. This is particularly true of reserve officers and this is where literally the colonel will take over the 03 Hearing Officer duty and (to compound his unrealized predicament) surround himself at the hearing with his staff, to show them how to cope with a situation none have met before.

The result: the *record* shows false standards, etc., etc. Any effort by the applicant's lawyer, if not most deferentially made, is met with a polite stare. It is like trying to influence a Ubangi Chief, in the presence of his courtiers.

All 03 Hearing Officers should be legal officers. No line officer can afford the time to become *knowledgeable* and justice cannot afford to permit such a man the privilege of boasting, "Yes, I've been a 03 Hearing Officer."

d. The *all-volunteer* army concept needs more than a ten million dollar Madison Avenue media approach—what is needed is emphasis on the just war *alone* plus patriotism approach. Youth, and the country, no longer accept the cliches: "My country right or wrong" or "Love America or Leave It" but will accept "I must do my part to see that my country is right, and, if changes are required, I'll help."

BIBLIOGRAPHY

1. Military Selective Service Act of 1967, 50 U.S. Code, App. § 462.
2.

Classification Picture February 28, 1970

Class	Number
Total	39,316,703
I-A and I-A-O	1,523,375
Single or married after August 26, 1965	
Examined and qualified	279,905
Not examined	68,737
Induction or examination postponed	13,030
Ordered for induction or examination	254,666
Pending reclassification	139,379
Personal appearance and appeals in process	58,691
Delinquents	32,946
Married on or before August 26, 1965	
Examined and qualified	5,871
Not examined	1,522
Induction or examination postponed	44
Ordered for induction or examination	302
Pending reclassification	600
Personal appearance and appeals in process	201
Delinquents	147
Nineteen years of age, born 1951	67,373
Twenty-six years and older with liability extended	157,599
Under 19 years of age	442,362
I-Y Qualified only in an emergency	3,360,945
I-C (Inducted)	484,886
I-C (Enlisted or commissioned)	2,376,802
I-O Not examined	7,667
I-O Examined and qualified	8,318
I-O Married, 19 to 26 years of age	709
I-W (At work)	8,983
I-W (Released)	10,990

I-D Members of a reserve component 924,387
I-S Statutory (College) 14,274
I-S Statutory (High School) 508,157
II-A Occupational deferment (except agricultural) 431,021
II-A Apprentice 56,932
II-C Agricultural deferment 22,829
II-S Student deferment 1,833,217
III-A Dependency deferment 4,194,121
IV-A Completed service; sole surviving son 3,393,042
IV-B Officials 85
IV-C Aliens 19,886
IV-D Ministers, divinity students 109,877
IV-F Not qualified 2,289,020
V-A Over age liability 17,737,180

When Dr. Tarr became Director he *streamlined* the above, among other things eliminating all the V-A (overage) men. Also, he soon thereafter destroyed their files.

When he was before the sub-committee last Fall [see footnote 12] he was asked by a committee member, a lawyer, "I have just a vague feeling that perhaps we might be doing ourselves a disservice by destroying the records, of eliminating the records, of registrants over 35 because it was my impression perhaps some circumstances in the future might require that we call on people above age 35 for one reason or another and, of course, these records wouldn't be available to us." [p. 12,487]

Dr. Tarr answered:

The reason I had to make a decision on this, and after exploring some of these records and talking with the people who maintain them, I have concluded that the records of these people are so far out of date, and it would be so difficult if we had to use people over thirty-five to correlate the records with the new information we gathered on them, that the existence of these records would actually be detrimental to an effort that we had to make in that short period of time, to recruit the people, for instance. [p. 12,487]

Dr. Tarr's new-style table reads:

Classification Picture

Class	Number
Total Current Registrants	21,908,000
I-A and I-A-O	2,017,000
Single or Married after August 26, 1965	
Examined and qualified 289,000	
Not examined 216,000	
Induction or examination postponed 9,000	
Ordered for induction or examination 127,000	

Pending reclassification	89,000
Personal appearances and appeals in process	59,000
Others	18,000
Married on or before August 26, 1965	7,000
19 years of age, born 1951, .1637.7(a)-(4)	663,000
26 years and older with extended liability	190,000
Under 19 years of age	350,000

I-Y Qualified only in an emergency	3,595,000
I-C Currently in the uniformed services	2,675,000
I-O Conscientious Objector	23,000
I-W (At Work)	9,000
I-W (Released)	12,000
I-D Members of a reserve component	953,000
I-S Statutory (College)	17,000
I-S Statutory (High School)	454,000
II-A Occupational deferment (except agriculture)	347,000
II-A Apprentice	50,000
II-C Agricultural deferment	22,000
II-S Student deferment	1,580,000
III-A Dependency deferment	4,118,000
IV-A Completed service; sole surviving son	3,656,000
IV-B Officials	*
IV-C Aliens	20,000
IV-D Ministers, divinity students	110,000
IV-F Not qualified	2,251,000

Figures as of August 31, 1970   * *Fewer than 1,000*

3. AR 40-501 (medical)
   AR 601-270 (moral)
   AR 604-10 (security)
   AR 635-89 (homo.)
   and many more

4. DoD 1300.6 (Defense)
   AR 635-20 (Army)
   AR 135-25 (A.Res.)
   AF 35-20 (Air F.)
   MCO 1306.16B (Mar.)
   BUPERSMAN 1860120 (Navy)
   COMDTINST 1900.2 (Coast G.)

5. There are no really reliable figures on this. The estimates, in the many dozen references, range from 10,000 to 60,000.

6. Suicide Prevention Center, Los Angeles County as reported in the *Los Angeles Times,* January 26, 1971:

> The suicide rate among young people in Los Angeles County has taken a sudden surge upward, the Suicide Prevention Center reported Monday.

For the first time in county history, the rate of suicides in the 20 to 29-year-old group is higher than the rates for the 30 to 39 and 40 to 49 age groups, Dr. Michael Peck, Director of Youth Studies at SPC, told a meeting on suicide here.

He said he first noted an upward shift in the rates for the young when analyzing the figures for 1968, which were fifty percent higher than 1967.

"At first I attempted to explain the change as being due to a cyclical fluctuation. But when the 1969 figures showed a 100 percent increase over 1968, I began to feel very uncomfortable with that explanation," Peck said.

7. Admiral Zumwalt, new Chief of Naval Operations has been widely quoted on this subject and many periodicals have shown pictures of the new hair styles permitted, etc.

8. The Army is going more slowly than the Navy; it is working on phasing into the professional army goal of the Administration.

9. *Selective Service News,* official monthly of the Selective Service System, December, 1970, and January, 1971.

10. Letter of John D. Alden, Executive Secretary, Engineering Manpower Commission to Subscribers of the EMC Information Service on Selective Service and Military Manpower Developments, dated February 16, 1971, enclosing his January 8, 1971, letter to Dr. Tarr and the latter's reply of January 25, 1971.

11. See No. 10 above.

12. Welsh v. United States 90 S.Ct. 1792 (1970). This case (1) decided that religious training and/or belief was not necessary for conscientious objection and (2) a Supreme Court justice [Mr. Harlan] wrote an opinion where, in addition to concurring in the result he pointed out, on pages 1798-1811, that the law was unconstitutional.

This decision has already caused many pending trial and Court of Appeal cases to be decided for the registrant, has obtained the release from prison of men who, the trial record showed, lost because their views were concededly sincere but philosophical, etc.

One of the interesting results has been that it, and it alone, gave Muhammed Ali (alias Cassius Clay) a new lease on life and enabled him to take on a $2,500,000.00 assignment in March, 1971.

The Congressional sub-committee asked Dr. Tarr "What is the status of Cassius Clay?" p. 12,529. His answer was too vague so the lawyer told him:

Would you put into the record the details and chronology of the *Cassius Clay* case. The general public is interested in this and the actions taken by the Federal Government?

(The following information was received for the record:)

Chronology of the Cassius Clay Case

Cassius Clay, SS No. 15-47-42-127.

Then followed a step by step account from February, 1961 to April 13, 1970, the last one reading:

Arguments were presented on this date [to the Court of Appeals for the Fifth Circuit] and decision will be forthcoming. (The last five entries shown above were reported on June 24, 1970 by the Criminal Division, Department of Justice.)

Then, in July his lawyers saw the applicability of *Welsh*. In 3 SSLR 43 (31 January 71) we read:

RECENT SUPREME COURT ACTIVITY

Review Activity

Between November 16, 1970 and January 12, 1971, the Supreme Court took the following action in pending cases:

1. Certiorari was granted on January 12, 1971 in no. 783, *Clay v. United States,* 3 SSLR 35, limited to question 4 of the petition:

> 4. Whether petitioner's convictions should be vacated in light of this Court's decision in Welsh v. United States, 398 U.S. 333, 3 SSLR 3001, because the denial to petitioner of a conscientious objector exemption may have been based on the Department of Justice's erroneous characterization of his objections to participation in war as "political and social" rather than "religious."

review—due process—validity of state director appeal procedure); *Gruca v. Sec'y of Army,* 3 SSLR 3372, ...F.2d. . . . (D.C.Cir. 1970) (conscientious objection—unconstitutional ground for denial); no. 1204, *Haifley v. United States,* 3 SSLR 3418, 432 F.2d 1064 (10th Cir. 1970) (conscientious objection—refusal to reopen after issuance of induction order—preinduction physical examination); no. 6411, *Hosmer v. United States,* 3 SSLR. . . .,. . . .F.2d . . . . (no. 7639, 1st Cir. Dec. 4, 1970) (right to counsel at personal appearance); no. 1016, *Jones v. United States,* 3 SSLR 3170, 431 F.2d 619 (9th Cir. 1970) (failure to report for induction—conscientious objection—right to exemption under *Welsh*); no. 6390, *Lloyd v. United States,* 3 SSLR 3160, *opp. modified,* 3 SSLR . . . ., ...F.2d. . . . (9th Cir. 1970) (conscientious objection)

Late editorial note: Subsequently, the Supreme Court reversed Clay's conviction 8-0, June 28, 1971, 91 S.Ct., 2068.

13. Full comment of the Central Committee for Conscientious Objectors. *Draft Counselor's Newsletter,* January, 1971. Note the restrained language.

The 1971 Selective Service Brochures: A Review

After nearly three decades of a Selective Service System under General Hershey that did its best to keep men from learning their options and rights, it is hard not to praise any serious effort by Selective Service to explain the draft in simple language, in enough detail to let men plan their lives with some awareness of their choices, and with recognition of the non-military as well as the military alternatives. "Perspective on the Draft" and three accompanying booklets entitled "C.O.," "The Lottery," and "Hardship Deferments," as well as a condensation of "Perspective" called "If You're Asked," are the first real steps in that direction to be issued under the directorship of Dr. Curtis W. Tarr.

The motive behind them may merit applause. But the booklets themselves must be given failing grades. They are recommended to draft counselors for reference only, as examples of Selective Service's notion of "basic draft facts" and as a warning to expect misinformed counselees. On at least three grounds, they cannot be recommended for distribution through responsible draft counseling centers in their present form. (This review is based on the second, and presumably final, text supplied by National Headquarters in a compilation headed "The 1971 Selective Service Brochures." Some counseling centers have received an earlier, and even worse, first edition.)

First, the booklets gloss over the shortcomings of Selective Service personnel and in the process give advice that can harm. "Perspective" tells 18-year-olds filling out the Classification Questionnaire who want more information about the classifications for which they may qualify: "Your local board will furnish you with details concerning such classifications." And "C.O." concludes, "Registrants who have further questions about how to claim C.O. status should seek the help and advice of a local board executive secretary." On top of that, the booklets don't contain even a hint that one might consult any other adviser: not only are draft counseling centers left unmentioned, but it isn't suggested that one can consult a clergyman or a school counselor. "Perspective" does recommend the precaution of using certified mail, but doesn't say that it is important to put all requests in writing, to save copies, and to summarize all personal contacts in writing soon afterwards; evidently the post office is unreliable but one can trust his friendly draft board always to protect his rights. On the other hand, "Perspective" deserves credit for warning that, "the Government appeal agent does not act as your attorney" and that "information you give him is not confidential, since he also advises the local board."

Second, the booklets omit huge amounts of essential information and don't suggest any other sources. "Perspective" says that appeals are aided by submission of "any pertinent information," but gives no ideas about the kinds of evidence needed. "Hardship Deferments" has a section on documentation which makes some good suggestions, but "C.O." doesn't even mention supporting letters. The section on personal appearances manages not to discuss their purpose, the ways to prepare for them, their duration, the procedures followed during them, or the steps to take afterward. The slight discussion of pre-induction physical examinations makes no reference to supplying medical evidence of disqualifying conditions, and doesn't mention the steps to take if the results are unsatisfactory. One could go on and on.

Third, all the booklets have serious inaccuracies, as well as many of the minor errors that tell you they were prepared by new, inexperienced employees. Among the significant errors: Two examples of circumstances that merit reopening are given—"serious injury" and "sudden family hardship." The first is a curious example, since local boards seem never to reopen a classification on the basis of medical evidence, unless so strong that it results in immediate disqualification without a physical. And the family hardship need not be "sudden," nor need one supply evidence of a "changed situation" to get a reopening before an induction order is issued. Though a man is supposed to notify the board within 10 days of any changes that could affect his classification (Reg. 1641.7), all that is needed for reopening is "nonfrivolous allegations of facts that have not previously been considered by his Board, and that, if true, would be sufficient under regulation or statute to warrant granting the requested classification . . . unless the truth of these new allegations is conclusively refuted by other reliable information in the file." (*U.S. v. Mulloy*, 3 SSLR 3011; LBM 111).

14. *The Reporter*, 28(1):1-2, January, 1971.
15. See No. 4.
16. Conversations with this writer in Israel, February, 1971.
17. Essential part of English National Service Act, 1948 (C. 64) s. 17.

APPENDIX B

HALSBURY'S
STATUTES OF ENGLAND
SECOND EDITION
EDITOR-IN-CHIEF
SIR ROLAND BURROWS, K.C.
RECORDER OF CAMBRIDGE
VOLUME 22
ROYAL FORCES
SALE OF GOODS AND HIRE PURCHASE
SALE OF LAND
SAVINGS BANKS
SET OFF AND COUNTERCLAIM
LONDON
BUTTERWORTH & CO. (PUBLISHERS) LTD.
BELL YARD, TEMPLE BAR, W.C.2.
1950
National Service Act, 1948 (c. 64), s. 17

Conscientious Objectors

17. Registration in register of conscientious objectors.—(1) If any person subject to registration claims that he conscientiously objects—

(a) to being registered in the military service register, or

(b) to performing military service, or

(c) to performing combatant duties,

he may, on furnishing the prescribed particulars about himself, apply in the prescribed manner to be registered as a conscientious objector in a special register to be kept by the Minister (in this Part of this Act referred to as *the register of conscientious objectors*):

Provided that where, in the case of a person who has been medically examined under section eight of this Act, such an application is made more than two days after the completion of his medical examination, the Minister shall dismiss the application unless he is satisfied, having regard to the grounds on which the application is made, that the making thereof has not been unreasonably delayed.

(2) Where any person applies in accordance with the last foregoing subsection to be registered in the register of conscientious objectors, he shall, unless his application is dismissed in accordance with the proviso to that subsection be provisionally registered in that register.

(3) A person who has been provisionally registered in the register of conscientious objectors shall within the prescribed period and in the prescribed manner, make to a local tribunal constituted under the Fourth Schedule to this Act an application stating to which of the matters mentioned in paragraphs (a) to (c) of subsection (1) of this section he conscientiously objects, and if he fails to do so the Minister shall remove his name from the register of conscientious objectors.

(4) An applicant for registration as a conscientious objector who is aggrieved by any order of a local tribunal and the Minister, if he considers it necessary, may, within the prescribed time and in the prescribed manner, appeal to the appellate tribunal constituted under the Fourth Schedule to this Act, and the decision of the appellate tribunal shall be final.

(5) The Minister or any person authorised by him shall be entitled to be heard on any application or appeal to a tribunal under this section.

(6) A local tribunal, if satisfied, upon an application duly made to it under this section, or the appellate tribunal is satisfied on appeal, that the ground upon which the application was made is established shall by order direct either—

(a) that the applicant shall without conditions be re-registered in the register of conscientious objectors; or

(b) that he shall be conditionally registered in that register until the end of a period of (eighteen months) and sixty days, the condition being that he must until the end of that period undertake work specified by the tribunal, of a civil character and under civilian control, and

(i) submit himself to such medical examination at such place and time as the Minister may direct for the purpose of ascertaining the applicant's fitness for that work;

(ii) undergo such training provided or approved by the

Minister as the Minister may direct for the purpose of fitting the applicant for that work;

and that at the end of that period he shall be registered in that register without conditions; or

(c) that he shall be registered in that register as a person liable or prospectively liable under this Part of this Act to be called up for service but to be employed only in non-combatant duties;

but, if not so satisfied, shall by order direct that his name shall be removed from the register of conscientious objectors:

Provided that in relation to any person who, by reason of his age, has not yet become liable under this Part of this Act to be called up for service, any condition imposed under paragraph (b) of this subsection shall be suspended until he attains the age of eighteen.

(7) The Minister may provisionally register in the register of conscientious objectors any person subject to registration, notwithstanding that he has refused or failed to make any application in that behalf, if in the Minister's opinion there are reasonable grounds for thinking that he is a conscientious objector, and the Minister may refer the case of that person to a local tribunal; and thereupon the provisions of this section shall have effect in relation to that person as if the necessary applications had been made by him, and references in this section to the *applicant* shall be deemed to include references to him.

(8) Any person unconditionally registered in the register of conscientious objectors by virtue of paragraph (a) of subsection (6) of this section or conditionally registered therein by virtue of paragraph (b) of that subsection shall not be liable to be called up for service so long as he is so registered.

(9) The Service Authorities shall make arrangements for securing that, where a person registered in the register of conscientious objectors by virtue of paragraph (c) of subsection (6) of this section as a person liable or prospectively liable under this Part of this Act to be called up for service but to be employed only in non-combatant duties is called up for service under this Part of this Act, he shall, during the period for which he serves by virtue of being so called up, be employed only in such duties.

(10) If, while a person is conditionally registered in the register of conscientious objectors, any change occurs in the particulars about him registered in that register, he shall forthwith notify the change to the Minister in the prescribed manner, and if he fails to do so shall be liable on summary conviction to a fine not exceeding five pounds. [132]

NOTES

This section reproduces s. 5 (except for sub-s. (8)) of the National Service (Armed Forces) Act, 1939 (c. 81), as amended by the National Service Act, 1941 (c. 15), s. 6 (1), (3) and Schedule, the National Service Act, 1942 (c. 3), s. 1 (3) and Schedule, the National Service Act, 1947 (c. 31), s. 17 (1), (2) and Third Schedule.

The words in square brackets were substituted for *twelve months* by the National Service (Amendment) Act, 1948, (c. 6) s. 1 (2).

Definitions. For *Minister, prescribed, conditionally registered* and *Service Authorities,* see s. 34 (1), p. 74, *post.*

Regulations under this section. National Service (Miscellaneous) Regulations, 1948, S.I. 1948 No. 2683, Part VII. For general provisions concerning regulations, see s. 32, p. 73, *post.*

Sub-s. (1).

Person subject to registration. For the construction of references to persons so subject, see ss. 6 (2), 10 (2), pp. 47, 53, *ante.*

Military service register. See s. 7 (4) (a), p. 48, *ante.*

Prescribed particulars; prescribed manner. See the National Service (Miscellaneous) Regulations, 1948, S.I. 1948 No. 2683, regs. 16, 17.

18. 32 C.F.R. Paragraph 1632.14
SSS Form No. 252.
19. The *Los Angeles Free Press* has a paid circulation of about 100,000. It has carried the following ads for a long period of time (one-third of a long list):

Los Angeles Free Press

DRAFT

FEEL THE DRAFT?

Venice Draft Information Service, 73 Market St., Rm. 2, Venice. Mon., Tues., Wed., Thurs. 7:30-10 p.m. Sat. 1-5 p.m. Call 399-5812: We need draft counselors and other volunteer help. Attorneys Mon. & Wed.

MILITARY COUNSELING

For GI counseling, legal aid, conscientious objection; or attorney referrals, contact Pacific Counseling Service at 514 West Adams Boulevard, Los Angeles, California 90007. Phone (213) 748-4662, 1924 Island Ave., San Diego, California 92102 (714) 239-2119. 24 hr. answering service.

DRAFT, MILITARY AND LEGAL COUNSELING is now available at the NORTH HOLLYWOOD FREE CLINIC, 5224 Lankershim Bl., every Tues., Thurs., Fri. 7-10 p.m. or by appt. Strictly confidential.

FREE DRAFT counseling San Fernando Valley. Mon. and Wed. 7-10 p.m. The Third Eye, 17150 Ventura Blvd. Call Help Line at 349-lawyer trained counselors.

HELP for additional information. Sponsored by Valley HelpLine

Even slick publications of national standing (as well as the more easily forgiven dailies) are not immune from spreading error. For example, *McCalls,* October, 1970, had a lengthy article entitled "I am a draft counselor" that would lead the reader to believe her Selective Service System registrant soon must present his deferment claims to the army! If he waits for them he will find deaf ears.

The Army has certain clear grounds for deferment. These are allowed not only for the benefit of the draftees, but to save the military the expense and trouble of training men who cannot or will not, for some reason, be able to serve. A skilled draft counselor helps a man file his claim for deferment according to the Army regulations that cover it. And he acts as a watchdog over procedural errors made by local boards—a boy drafted out of high school, for instance, because someone made a mistake.

20. *Time,* February 8, 1971, page 48, relates a series of such denials including:

Aronson introduced a newspaper clipping about a whorehouse that had such a phone and added that to reach client McLemore's military attorney he had had to place 233 calls to the military switchboard —only four of which ultimately got through to the right man. With all of the obstacles, L.M.D.C. lawyers saw McLemore for the first time only one hour before going into the courtroom.

21. Personal experiences of the author, plus dozens of reported court cases so showing, both embodied in Supreme Court briefings.

Chapter 16

AGE OF AQUARIUS

FRANK LANTERMAN

O
N JULY 1, 1969, California reversed more than a century of
comparative disregard of the legal, civil and personal rights
of its mentally ill citizens.

With the enactment by the legislature of the Lanterman-
Petris-Short Act, we have completely restructured many long-
established, obsolete legal restraints that have for far too many
years characterized the involuntary treatment of the mentally disordered.

Passage of this bill did not come easily. The L-P-S Act is the
product of more than two years of intensive legislative study.

The study led to the *Dilemma of Mental Commitments*,
published by the Assembly Ways and Means Subcommittee on
Mental Health Services in 1966. This report and its recommendations were the basis for the new legislation. The report was
based on a thorough survey of mental health literature, exten-
sive observations of most of California's commitment courts, and
an analysis of the characteristics of 5,000 mentally disordered
patients in every psychiatric hospital in the state. This dilemma
report is now being used as a text in a Harvard Law course and
others. It is an understatement to say that it has attracted medical, legal and judicial attention nationally.

For those of you who may not be totally familiar with L-P-S,
I would like to take a few minutes to briefly discuss the major
provisions of the L-P-S Act.

The thrust of the act is to promote voluntary treatment for
the mentally disordered. The provisions for involuntary treatment have been written so that they will be the *last* resort rather
than the first, as was so often the case in the past.

In order to understand the new law and its overwhelming
support in both houses of the legislature, a look at California's
previous mental health system is necessary. For too many years

people assumed that a mentally disturbed individual would not admit to being *sick* and would not accept recommended treatment. Therefore, it was thought necessary to contain and restrain him so that he could not escape from treatment. This was sometimes justified on the grounds that "the individual will later recognize that it was all for his own good."

The legislature found this concept indefensible for two important reasons: first, there was no guarantee that the treatment given to this *captive patient* would actually improve his condition; and second, the restrictive methods used to hold a protesting patient for treatment too often created other social and personality problems which damaged his chances for improvement.

Not only was the philosophy underlying the old commitment process full of contradictions, but the day-to-day judicial *enforcement* mechanism of the system actually delayed treatment and violated individual freedoms and civil rights. In a study which is detailed in the assembly report, it was discovered that the average commitment hearing in California lasted 4.7 minutes! *Railroading* is a strong word, but if *railroading* means taking away a person's liberty for an indefinite period after a cursory examination in a crowded observation ward and a perfunctory commitment hearing lasting less than five minutes, then we were all too often guilty of *railroading* in the commitment court. Too often *due process* was sidetracked completely.

Uninformed community attitudes toward eccentric, unwanted and burdensome citizens, and the lack of available local mental health services were the main reasons which perpetuated this tragic disposition of more than 1,000 citizens every month, year after year.

The new L-P-S law has changed these old procedures and has provided communities with the ability to deal with serious mental problems. Since July 1, 1969, the implementation date of the new L-P-S Act, commitment courts in California have been virtually eliminated (excepting, of course, the criminally insane and the sexual psychopath commitments, which are not affected by the L-P-S provisions). In their place, the act provides for involuntary detention *only* when a person is a danger to himself or others, or gravely disabled, and even then, *only for brief, specifically limited periods of time.* In other words, voluntary services must be carefully ruled out before *involuntary* treatment can be imposed.

A person who, as a result of mental disorder, is a *danger to himself or others or gravely disabled* may be held for a 72-hour evaluation period. If, after a screening diagnosis by various specifically qualified multidisciplinary professionals, the person is still in the same condition at the end of three days' observation and will not accept help on a voluntary basis, the patient may be certified for an additional fourteen days of involuntary treatment. If he is no longer a danger to himself or others or gravely disabled at the completion of fourteen days, he must be released. The old law permitted *indefinite periods of involuntary treatment* for any one who was considered to be *in need of treatment, care, supervision, or restraint.*

If an individual has attempted or threatened suicide during the first seventeen days, he may be certified for one additional fourteen-day treatment period. After the second two weeks have elapsed, the patient must be released.

These time periods have been substantiated as optimum involuntary treatment periods. Professional opinion indicates that this is sufficient time to get most people through the crisis period and to a point where they will accept help voluntarily, preferably on an outpatient basis.

Dr. Werner Mendel, University of Southern California School of Medicine, after a rigorous study of 3,000 schizophrenic patients, stated, "Patients with mental illness cannot get well inside a hospital." (As Dr. Farabee of Kentucky has so eloquently said, "get them out of bed!") The legislature concurred and the new law asserts that people can be helped most after a minimum of personal dislocation and a rapid return to their own familiar environment.

The legislature did recognize, however, that longer involuntary detention may sometimes be justified on the basis of public safety. For this reason, the law also establishes additional 90-day periods of involuntary care for those persons who, immediately prior to or during the first seventeen days of screening and treatment, have shown themselves to be *overtly* dangerous to others. This fact of overt danger must be proven in a court of law and if no further evidence of physical danger exists after the termination of 90 days, the person must be released.

The fear has been expressed that many *potentially* dangerous persons would not meet the criteria under the law and would be released at the end of seventeen days. We are speaking here of a patient's right to liberty. We have already kept this person involuntarily for up to seventeen days on the strength of clinical opinions. Any additional involuntary treatment must be justified in court on the basis of public safety.

The Ways and Means Subcommittee on Mental Health Services chose not to leave the determination to hold a person for 90 days to medical discretion. Why? Because psychiatry is not an exact science with precise predictive tools. Therefore, physical evidence of *danger to others* must be proven in a court of law before the patient can be held for an additional 90 days. The legislature *does not sanction preventive jailing* of those who have committed no crime.

The category of *danger to self* was purposely excluded from the 90-day post certification procedure. In the research conducted by the subcommittee, we found no evidence to support the value of prolonged hospitalization for the suicidal person. In fact, we found that lengthy involuntary treatment may be the worst form of therapy. Testimony from the Los Angeles Suicide Prevention Center indicated that intensive treatment during the short crisis period is the most effective. We must also face the fact that there is no way to prevent a person from taking his life if he is determined to do so.

Under the old law, a person brought in on a 72-hour hold often received only a cursory examination before being brought before a commitment court and sent to a state hospital. By the time the individual received any treatment his condition was often worse than it was when he was apprehended. The new treatment periods allow for immediate and intensive treatment from the moment the person enters the door. This is the intent of the act. In addition, the new evaluation period includes an investigation of alternatives to involuntary care, a procedure rarely followed during the old perfunctory commitment hearings.

The provision for medical rather than judicial 14-day certification stems from recommendations by the medical profession. We felt that the value of rapid and continuous help outweighed the benefits of automatic, cursory judicial review. But, in order to protect the patient, the new law includes a provision for immediate jury trial upon the request of the patient.

The L-P-S Act also contains a provision for *mandatory prepetition screening*. The effectiveness of professional screening is shown in the experience with the nonpsychotic seniles. In the subcommittee's hospital survey, it was shown that 20 percent of persons committed were over 65. Yet the San Francisco Geriatric Screening Unit, which vigorously explores alternatives to commitment of the aged, has reduced geriatric commitments in that city from over 400 per year in 1963 to four in 1967.

I have discussed the categories of danger to self and others, but I have not described the provisions for the gravely disabled person, that is, someone who is unable to care for his basic bodily needs of food, clothing and shelter. If during the 17-day treatment period, an individual is identified by mental health professionals as being gravely disabled, then a new *conservatorship procedure* is used. This procedure requires a thorough examination of the patient's condition and the appointment of an appropriate conservator who will determine the most beneficial placement of this individual. Conservatorship is for a one-year period which terminates automatically unless renewed. The law emphasizes community treatment rather than state institutionalization for such persons.

One major side effect of state hospitalization has been the traumatic stigma which has long separated the mental patient from all other citizens. Under previous law both voluntary and involuntary mental patients suffered serious legal disabilities. In fact, the mental patient was historically subject to *seven* more legal disabilities than a *convicted felon*. The act abolishes all such automatic disabilities. (My questions to Dr. Lowry in our Ways and Means Committee hearing on these statutory deprivations started the study resolution in 1966.)

The law also guarantees legal and civil rights long denied mental patients receiving *involuntary* treatment including the right: (1) to have reasonable access to telephones, both to make and receive personal and confidential calls; (2) to have access to letter writing materials, including stamps, and to mail and receive unopened correspondence; (3) to refuse shock treatment, and (4) to refuse lobotomy.

Patient's rights under provisions of the act may be denied only for good cause and when denied this must be entered into the person's treatment record and made available for official review. We feel this is a sound provision.

Finally, the act requires confidentiality of records so that mentally ill persons will not be haunted for a lifetime by unauthorized and unnecessary exposure of their medical histories. Minor adjustments are now being considered in order to meet some problems of law enforcement with the strict confidentiality provisions.

In addition to commitment reform, the law provides for an orderly transition from a large institutional mental health program to one centered in local communities nearest to the home of the patient.

Through the unification of the state and local mental health budgets and a new 90 percent state—10 percent local financing formula, the act links previously separate programs, creates a program budget, and provides strong fiscal incentives for the expansion of local programs.

In January, 1967, there were 41 local mental health centers treating 128,000 patients with the state paying $15 million of the cost. Today, there are 53 centers treating in excess of 160,000 patients, and the state has budgeted over $75 million for local programs.

The new act requires each county to develop a county Short-Doyle plan for the organization of all mental health resources. The county Short-Doyle plan is the planning mechanism for the allocation of funds for services to the mentally disordered whether they are served locally or in the state hospital.

In addition, the legislature recognizes the need for priorities in the distribution of county and state mental health dollars. Each county Short-Doyle plan must include priorities for developing local services. To aid the counties and the state in developing mental health priorities, five-year mental health service plans must be prepared by local and state government.

The major goal of this legislation is to foster community services and local decision making regarding the treatment needs of county citizens. The state remains the senior partner in financing mental health services and setting standards, but local government is now enabled to "relate the trouble and the cure to the entire web of social and personal relationships in which the individual is caught."

The concept of care expressed in the principles embodied in the L-P-S Act has aroused a widespread interest, hope and concern across the nation. California is encouraged that sister states have also taken enlightened legislative action. A nationwide poll shows that more than 66 percent of the sample interviewed favored abolishment of the involuntary commitment of the mentally ill.

I am not trying to suggest that there is uncontested acceptance of this massive reform. But I can say without hesitation that the *doubting Thomases* are fading rapidly. Many have joined the ranks of supporters. Two-thirds approval nationwide of the humanitarian principles of protection and care for the mentally ill is progress.

We have already survived one major challenge when the state supreme court ruled last year that L-P-S was constitutional. Our studious efforts to protect the dignity and civil rights of our mentally ill citizens must be sustained and perfected.

We are deeply indebted to the attorney general's office and his most able and competent deputy, Jan Stevens, whose thorough and persuasive presentation to the supreme court was instrumental in upholding and preserving the constitutional legal status of L-P-S.

We have also survived the repeated challenges of the California State Employees Association, whose management has speculated that the L-P-S Act might eventually mean the end of a state hospital system. I do not agree! The state hospital system *will continue* to function as a resource, but there will be fewer hospitals as some are phased out as obsolete, and those that remain will provide higher standards of care only for patients who require protracted institutional treatment. We cannot justify the expense of keeping open a massive chain of partially filled state hospitals. Hospital employees should be retained on the payroll only at a level of improved staffing standards in relationship to the nature of the patient load.

In order to assure an objective evaluation of this comprehensive new program, the assembly in conjunction with a private research corporation, is conducting a two year *before and after* study under a research grant from the National Institute of Mental Health. The research firm collected data and observed the mental health system in California several months in advance of the implementation date of the program and is continuing to evaluate the law through August of this year. This type of study should provide us an excellent basis for comparing the old system against the new and to examine L-P-S and its strengths and weaknesses.

We are determined that the L-P-S Act shall be improved and perfected. In fact, we are now in the midst of considering recommendations from all over the state to refine the law where necessary, keeping in mind it is only in its second year of operation. As during the past two years, I have introduced a bill to *clean up* the minor mechanical and technical problems that are bound to occur when a long-established system is entirely restructured. During this refining process we are continuing to consult with all interested agencies and individuals. The California Conference of Judges, the Conference of Local Mental Health Directors, the California Mental Health Association, the Public Guardians Association, CSAC, and various county administrators must be singled out for their constructive suggestions. I also want to express my deep appreciation to Dr. Lowry and his legal staff of the Department of Mental Hygiene who have spent so many long hours with us during the drafting and revision sessions.

In summary, there is substantial progress being made in our programs for the mentally ill in California. It is a time of transition, of advances in research, of improved services and particularly in the development of comprehensive, locally-based community programs through a state-community partnership. We are struggling to iron out the problems of cash flow and equity between counties.

We have come a long way since 1851 when the California State Legislature appropriated the funds for establishment of Stockton State Hospital—the first mental institution west of the Rocky Mountains. We have come a long way from the archaic era of locked wards and public attitudes which stigmatized the mentally ill and retarded as something evil, possessed and unclean, to be put away in remote restraint, removed from reality.

We are determined to continue to make progress in full realization of our continuing responsibility. Patience and forebearance are the watchwords, so that we may provide to the fullest extent possible care and treatment for those who have nowhere else to turn.

Chapter 17

THE PSYCHOLOGICAL HEALTH OF THE CITY TODAY

ALFRED AUERBACK, M.D.

T HE HISTORY of cities is intimately related to the history of civilization. Man's progress in industry, commerce, religion, education, and the arts is closely entwined with the city. The city came into being when the solitary hunter or farmer, threatened by predators from the outside, sought security in living with his fellows. From the beginning the city provided protection from external dangers, a marketplace, and a center for religious purposes. The security the city provided gave man a sense of freedom and the opportunity to turn his energies to activities other than defense.

The explosive urbanization of the past half-century has occurred without much planning and with the individual less and less in control of his surroundings. Today urban life no longer provides a sense of belonging. As Toynbee has said: "The most insecure places in the present day world are no longer the surviving jungles and deserts; they are the urban slums. The slum-dwelling human gangster has become a more formidable predator on urbanized man than the lions and tigers that are preserved behind bars in the city's zoo."[1] He sums up life in the city today as follows: "Man is paying for having overcome external dangers by becoming a still greater danger to himself. He is the victim of his triumphant science, technology and organization. Technology has inflated the material setting of human life to an inhuman scale. Man is being dwarfed by his apparatus and stifled by his numbers, and this heavy physical pressure on the individual is inflicting a severe psychic distress. The problem of defense in Megalopolis is the problem of how to rehumanize life when it has to be lived in a man-made infinity of people, buildings and streets."[2]

270

Social Changes in the City

The city initially grew around a central core where increasing numbers of people gathering together provided both the work force and the customers for business and industry. As the cities grew, those residents who could moved to the periphery. Those unable to move remained in the central core. The vacated homes were quickly filled by the incoming groups, immigrants from other countries or elsewhere within the country. The developing industry and businesses utilized the unskilled by providing training which permitted them to fit into the civic structure. As they became more skilled and their children better educated, they were able to move upwards in the social scale. They in turn abandoned the central city leaving it to the ever-continuing flow of newcomers who took their places.

Processing of raw materials into finished products provided employment for the unskilled newcomers. The shift from manufacturing to service industries today requires higher skills and better education; the untrained, unskilled newcomers now find fewer and fewer work opportunities. Since World War II there has been a major movement of the black population in the United States from the south to the northern cities. Although blacks constitute only 10 percent of the American population, they now represent large numbers in the city and often constitute a majority of the city population. While some have prospered and have become upwardly mobile, many have found that their limited education would not equip them for the technological society.

The rapid influx of blacks into the cities of the past two decades has brought serious problems involving employment, housing and education. The demands of the black population for equal rights and opportunities have brought them into conflict with many of the white population. This racial unrest has been accentuated by the presence of other minority groups, Mexican-American, Puerto Rican, American Indian and in some communities, Chinese and Japanese minorities. Racism has resulted from the tension between the white and nonwhite groups. Racial riots have developed, reflecting a breakdown in communication and the inability of the city and its citizens to cope with the problems of the minority groups.

Within the central city a progressive, physical deterioration has taken place over the years, and today much of it constitutes the ghetto and the slums. Here are increasingly larger concentrations of the poor, the old, the alienated youth, and the racial minorities; people whose poverty produces insecurity, inferiority, irritability and feelings of helplessness. Life in the ghetto is colored by crime, social unrest, discontent, despair, profound unhappiness and considerable experience with prejudice. The immense pressures from this large number of underprivileged citizens, with their attendant civic and social problems, have forced the city to make some efforts to correct the situation. This has produced a steady increase in tax burdens which in turn has led to mounting resentment on the part of the taxpayers.

Financial Problems of the Cities

In the past the cities had political and financial strengths that no longer exist. In 1932 local governments collected more taxes than state and federal governments combined; in that year 52 percent of the taxes were collected at the local level. Thirty years later this had dropped to 7 percent and the percentage has decreased steadily since. During this same period much of the middle class and many businesses had moved out of the city, into the suburbs, removing substantial income from the city's tax rolls. This loss of population has reduced the city's political representation at state and federal levels.

Decisions having a vital impact on the well-being of the city are now made at distant points by individuals or groups who have no personal involvement with the city. In the state legislatures the city has a steadily decreasing political voice. The federal government closes a shipyard, hospital, military base, or agency without consulting the civic administration. National corporations can close manufacturing plants or regional offices, throwing hundreds or even thousands of persons out of work. Too often the city finds itself impotent in influencing decisions crucial to its health and viability.

Today, the cities find themselves in a unique position—most are becoming bankrupt. They are confronted by a loss of revenues at a time when the costs of their operation are rapidly rising. Welfare and medical services consume monies that would otherwise go to vital services such as public safety, education and transportation. Twenty years ago the city of New York had an annual budget of one billion dollars to finance all its services. Today that amount does not meet the needs of the one in seven who are on relief in that city. Between 1965 and summer 1971, the number of people on welfare in the United States almost doubled from 7.7 million to 14.2 million.[3] The financial cost rose from 5.3 to 16.3 billion dollars. Percentage-wise the number of people on welfare has increased faster than the rate of population growth.

Despite the astronomical amounts of money being spent, there is no evidence to indicate that it has been anything more than a stop-gap arrangement. Welfare payments have neither helped the underprivileged out of their dependent role nor brought them into the mainstream of the economic system. While some welfare recipients feel demeaned, others have come to consider it a right. Taxpayers confronted by a never-ending financial drain with no apparent alternative solution, are becoming increasingly resistant. If present trends continue, it is anticipated that by 1975, 8 percent of the population will be on welfare at an annual cost of 25 billion dollars.

One of the most disturbing aspects of the welfare problem is the increasing cost of assisting families with dependent children. At the present time, some nine million people in the United States are on relief because of dependent children. This represents 69 percent of all people on welfare and 54 percent of all welfare costs. The financial costs may be staggering, but the psychological implications are even more troublesome. Millions of children are growing up in homes that are financially impoverished, often unable to provide adequate nutrition or shelter. This leads to physical, emotional, and mental impairment. In most cases the children are growing up in broken homes, with no comprehension of a healthy family structure, nor the role of adequate parents. Efforts to provide compensatory education have proven to be of limited value. There is no evidence that the large sums of money being spent are in any measure preparing these children for productive lives as adults.

Changes in the Physical Environment

The cities have undergone a dramatic transformation with a building boom to provide working space and housing for the ever-expanding population. Skyscrapers, bridges, freeways and shopping plazas are hailed as measures of civic progress. Most of this growth is without unified plan, as the city spreads out to engulf the land around it. Behind the glossy face of the city, behind the glass, marble, and concrete, lie the slums; the city is a *goodly apple rotten at the heart.* Surrounded by steel and concrete the heart of the city is being choked to death. Freeways and expressways bisect the city, cutting it into discontinuous segments. Automotive traffic brings air and noise pollution. Cross-town automobile travel takes the same length of time as horse travel, half a century ago.

The deteriorating, blighted areas of central city slums constitute the breeding places of social-psychopathology, of physical and mental illness, of discontent, turmoil and unhappiness. The high rates of death, divorce, delinquency, suicide, unemployment, illegitimacy, alcoholism and venereal disease are part of an endless list of social and medical disorders.

Efforts to improve the slums have not yet been successful. Public housing and urban renewal have so far proven to be a disappointment; more living quarters for the poor have been destroyed than replaced. The pent-up fury of the disaffected, neglected and dispossessed now finds more frequent expression in crime, riots, bombings, demonstrations, arson and other ways of striking back at the city, at its banks and businesses, and too often at the ghetto itself.

Life in the city today brings increasing strain and noxious stimuli. The ever-increasing populace brings larger numbers of people living and working more closely together, subjecting them to crowding, noise pollution, air pollution and loss of privacy. Studies of animals living under crowded conditions show a disintegration of their personal relationships, and a generalized social disorganization. Human crowding produces irritability, suspicion, anger and violence.

The absence of personal privacy and the constant stimuli impinging on the individual impairs his sense of identity. Much of his energy is devoted to defending himself against these outside pressures. Withdrawal, detachment, anger or violence become coping mechanisms for some; others turn to alcohol or drugs as an attempt to handle stress. Selye's studies on stress have shown how constant noxious stimuli give rise to physical and psychological illness.[4] Urban life today is accompanied by increasing anxiety, depression and psychosomatic illness.

Doxiadis stated that the city of the past had a definite simple structure which allowed man, as an inhabitant, to comprehend it easily, to move about without difficulty in a way that served all his needs, and to administer it properly. According to Doxiadis the dimensions and structure of today's cities are beyond the comprehension of the individual citizen. He is unable to grasp their totality. His area of involvement rarely extends beyond his immediate environment. He continues, "It is no longer easy for man to comprehend, to live in, or to administer the contemporary city, because it has grown out of the human scale, grown out of control."[5]

Youth in the City

City life imposes tremendous strains on the family and the child. The American family has become highly mobile; many families have lost their roots. More and more society is based on temporary relationships; the extended family no longer exists. Grandparents, uncles, aunts, and cousins, who formerly supplied support, continuity, and a sense of family belonging, no longer live close at hand. The role of the family is in profound transition and demands increasing flexibility and ability to adapt to rapidly changing situations. More and more, material possessions substitute for emotional interaction. Increasingly mothers go to work, sometimes to buy material comforts, but often to keep the family financially viable. Many children are cared for by baby-sitters, family friends or the staff of a child care center. There is limited contact with parents giving rise to a decrease in parental influence and parental control, and an increase of anxieties and concerns in the child about his personal identity, and place in the world.

Between five and six million youngsters are growing up in single parent families. The 1970 United States census indicated that 10.9 percent of white children and 39.5 percent of nonwhite children have one or both parents missing. In most cases the parent is the mother, divorced or deserted, who attempts to support and raise a family by herself. Children raised in the home without a father are too often ill-equipped to make good marital adjustments. The boy has anxieties about his male identity, while the girl without a father may develop a distorted understanding of the male role. The seeds for psychological, sociological and medical disorders are planted during these turbulent years.

Outside the home, children are confronted by a threatening world. This is the second generation growing up in the shadow of the atomic bomb. Children hear talk about the population explosion, air pollution, water pollution, overuse of pesticides and the possibility that man may soon destroy himself. An unpopular war has existed for the past decade. Youth are confronted by an uncertain world and wonder if they will find a place for themselves when they are adults. Religion no longer provides answers and many turn to astrology, mysticism, or escape through drugs. Technology, which at one time promised happiness through its accomplishments, appears to have failed. Youth are increasingly aware of injustice, of poverty in a land of plenty, of exploitation, and above all the fact that they have little or no power to bring about change.

The city itself evinces little interest in its youth. Few cities offer much in the way of recreational facilities; most youngsters find their playgrounds in the street, where they compete with the automotive traffic. Demands for change on the part of youth find a cold reception by the civic establishment. There are inadequate outlets provided for the energy and enthusiasm of youth. Now that eighteen-year-olds are permitted to vote, there may be a change. Up to this point, few youngsters have been able to involve themselves at the civic level. Basically they have felt alienated and have been cut-off, without voice or power.

In the past, schools offered refuge from urban stress. Education held the promise of opening doors to a secure future. However, that promise is blurred today. There is no certainty that the education provided youth today equips them for the world of tomorrow. Teaching is often related to the past rather than the needs of the present and the future. Often the school itself is a physical relic of the past, 30 to 50 years old, dilapidated, with outmoded equipment, and reflecting the wear and tear of thousands of youngsters. In some schools, particularly in the ghetto areas, there may be a turnover of half the student body during the school year. The teaching profession is also going through its own turbulence. At the present time there is a surplus of teachers with steadily decreasing job opportunities. Students and the public hold teachers in less esteem; many teachers have a diminished sense of accomplishment in conducting their classes.

Within recent years schools and the educational system generally have found themselves under increasing attack. Children, teachers, and administrators now find themselves pawns in power struggles over school integration, busing, sex education and the provision of quality education. Parents are becoming increasingly angry and discontented with the education their children receive. They now demand more voice in the operation of schools. Their displeasure finds expression in voting down bond issues to improve schools or the educational systems. Limited finances have forced many schools to increase class sizes, reduce curricula, eliminate remedial courses, and curtail the school term. Schools may be firetraps or vulnerable to earthquakes but often the taxpayers refuse to replace them, ignoring the hazards they represent to children.

In the early 1970's schools manifest a level of turmoil hitherto unknown. Vandalism, assault on teachers and other students, even rape, are becoming commonplace. In the halls and schoolyards, drugs are readily and increasingly available. Peer pressure leads to drug experimentation, and for some, addiction. The ever-increasing number of uneducated, poorly-educated, or poorly motivated youngsters disrupts the school and lowers the general level of education for all. Integration of the schools has been successful in some localities, but less so in others. Puberty comes earlier than in the past, with accompanying biological stresses.

At the same time society's economic demands for higher education maintain the adolescent in a dependent state which may extend into the adult years. For the lonely, the discontented, and the alienated, school is an unhappy experience. Many drop out of school. Others turn to drugs or alcohol as a means of escape. Childhood and adolescence particularly in the heart of the changing city are often not happy years. Too many children are subjected to changing homes, changing friends, changing schools, to the point where they feel that there is nothing permanent in their lives.

Psychiatric Illness in the City

The Mid-Town Manhattan Study revealed that nearly 25 percent of New York's population had serious psychological problems that required psychiatric help.[6] Most were not receiving this help. Broken homes, economic deprivation, poor physical and mental health, family friction and poor family relationships were significant factors in the lives of those individuals who subsequently developed some form of psychiatric illness. In New York, as well as in every other community that has been studied, the largest numbers of psychological disabilities come from the impoverished, deprived residents of the central city. While psychiatric illness is most concentrated in this sector, it can be found at all social levels. Mental illness, alcoholism, drug abuse, depressive reactions, mental retardation, school problems and psychosomatic illness do not respect social class; they are omnipresent.

In December, 1970, as chairman of the San Francisco Mental Health Advisory Board, I submitted a report on mental health services in that city. The report stated that it was impossible to give fixed numbers regarding psychiatric illness. The majority of people do not seek help due to fear, ignorance, or mistrust. Many of the mentally and emotionally disturbed are transient, coming from other parts of the country and unaware of health services available to them.

Through sampling techniques it was possible to estimate some dimensions of the problem. Probably one fifth of San Francisco's population have a need for psychiatric services. Currently 22,000 are seen annually in public mental health services; less than half that number of San Franciscans are treated by private practising psychiatrists each year. A recent survey revealed that the percentage of private psychiatric patients in different parts of the city had almost 100 percent correspondence with the population percentages.[7] The Mission District with 17.6 percent of San Francisco's population supplied 17 percent of private patients, the Sunset-Richmond (28 percent) had 24 percent of private patients, the North-East (18 percent) had 16 percent of private patients. There were two notable exceptions. Affluent Pacific Heights showed 180 percent overusage while the Hunters Point ghetto had marked underusage of private care, only 20 percent.

An estimated 48,000 San Franciscans have a drinking problem sufficient to interfere with their normal functioning. Hepatic cirrhosis, in nearly every case related to excessive drinking, results in death four times the national average. Suicide is the seventh cause of death in San Francisco, almost four times the national rate. It has been estimated that for every suicide, there are at least five and possibly ten suicidal attempts. Of the estimated 20,000 ambulatory mentally ill, mostly schizophrenic, about one quarter have an acute psychotic episode requiring attention at some time during the year. Approximately 18,000 children are mentally disturbed, representing 10 percent of the total population under age 18. The seriously disturbed youngsters manifest psychotic illness, delinquent behavior or acute crisis situations. It is believed that at least 35,000 more youngsters have problems that could be helped by some counselling service.

The past decade has seen a dramatic change in the nature of psychiatric illness, particularly in the categories characterized as personality and character disorders. These are neurotic reactions where the individual's emotional problems give rise to self-defeating behavior, often self-destructive and antisocial. The antisocial behavior is characterized by the excessive use of alcohol or drugs, deviant sexual behavior, delinquency, over-aggressiveness, vandalism and other forms of acting-out behavior. Most alarming has been the increasing use of drugs, particularly by adolescents and young adults. At an age when they should be developing directions for their lives, they have turned to drugs as a coping mechanism. San Francisco is estimated to have 7,000 heroin addicts. Its methadone treatment program for heroin addicts has recorded an 86 percent social rehabilitation rate for participants in this program. It is uncertain that such a high success rate can be maintained as the program is enlarged.

The methadone program in San Francisco is currently being tripled and it is planned to further this expansion in view of its apparent success up to this time. Admittedly, methadone maintenance as a treatment leaves much to be desired, since it substitutes one addiction for another. At this time, it appears to be among the best treatments developed for the social rehabilitation of heroin addicts. The cost to the community through burglary, hold-ups, shoplifting and assault to obtain money to support the heroin habit is so excessive that any reduction in the actual number of addicts cannot help but bring about marked monetary savings. Additional benefits include a reduction in the need for police and custodial services, and a general lessening of community anxieties about these antisocial individuals.

Alcoholism is a disease that affects a remarkably high percentage of the urban population. Alcohol has always been used as a vehicle of escape from tension. It is a major cause of physical illness, early death, and family disruption. It has been estimated that the excessive use of alcohol by an individual adversely affects at least four others, including spouse, family, employer and friends. It is now recognized that children growing up in families where alcohol is used excessively are prone to develop serious psychiatric disorders in later years. While some cities provide minimal treatment for persons with alcoholic problems, most become involved with the police and the courts. Up to 50 percent of all arrests in the metropolitan areas are related to the excessive use of alcohol. Most traffic fatalities are related to excessive drinking. Where efforts are made to assist the alcoholic, a remarkably high percentage can be successfully returned to the community.

The incidence of psychiatric illness in New York and San Francisco is the same in communities throughout the country. All communities, large and small, show the same picture of psychopathology. There is no question that the dramatic changes in family structure and the ongoing impairment of parent-child relationships are intimately related to this high incidence of psychiatric disorder. Even when the community develops a system of care designed to deliver mental health services, it is not always successful. This arises from the fact that many of the individuals in need of mental health services are also suffering from other civic or social problems: poverty, discrimination, unemployment, inadequate education, transportation and housing difficulties, malnutrition, disenfranchisment, and above all, a sense of alienation from society.

Today medical and psychiatric services are beginning to meet in some degree the needs of these otherwise lost citizens. Most programs for improvement have failed because of an inability to recognize the social problems and an unwillingness to give the consumers more voice and involvement in those decisions that affect their lives. There is now a grudging acceptance by the urban power structure of the fact that mental and physical health involves not only the absence of disease but also the social well-being of the individual and of the groups in the community. This includes living conditions, working conditions, adequate nutrition, and recreational outlets. In the absence of these, good physical and mental health cannot exist. In particular, children require stability in their homes and in their environment if they are to develop the abilities that will equip them for productive lives in their adult years.

Violence in the City

Some degree of violence has always been associated with urban life. Now violence has escalated to the point where it threatens not only the physical well-being of the citizenry but the life of the city itself. This is related to two new developments. One is the increasing use of drugs and its impact on society. The second is the increasing resort to violence on the part of individuals who find that other methods of obtaining acceptance, employment, and equal opportunity have failed.

Only a few years ago the use of drugs was limited to a small segment of the urban population, primarily in the lower socioeconomic groups. Now drug abuse is present in all levels of society. Youngsters use it at a rate never seen before. For some it is a transient experimentation. For others, it represents a rebellion against parental demands and expectations or an escape from the uncertainties of life. Marijuana, LSD, amphetamines and barbiturates have had increasing use by children, adolescents, and young adults. Their use gives rise to antisocial behavior, violence, self-destruction, withdrawal or other acting-out behavior. However the most destructive drug is heroin. Heroin in itself does not produce antisocial behavior, but rather a feeling of inner tranquility. As an addictive drug it requires regular use at an average cost of perhaps $50 a day. To obtain this money, girls resort to prostitution or shoplifting. Men resort to armed robbery, burglary or the sale of drugs. In New York City at least 100,000 and perhaps as many as 200,000 persons are addicted to heroin. In San Francisco at least 7,000 heroin addicts prey on the public. The use of heroin is associated with a remarkably high death rate.

City life is no longer safe; assault or robbery on the streets have become commonplace. People are attacked, shot or stabbed for small amounts of money, sometimes for no apparent reason. Women experience purse-snatching, assault and rape. Sudden death on the street is a common event. Even the home is no longer safe; violent entry is on the increase. Fear is present everywhere. No one feels safe on the streets at night, even in his own neighborhood. Shopping downtown no longer interests the housewife because of the possible dangers. This hastens the physical and financial collapse of the business districts. On the street the stranger is treated with profound distrust. Homes and stores have become fortresses with guards, burglar alarms and loaded guns to repel the potential intruder. Suspicion and mistrust affect the city, and like a cancer, eat away at its spirit.

To a large degree, violence, assault and burglary are related to the search for money to maintain the heroin habit. However, once lawlessness becomes rampant, it feeds on itself. Respect for the individual and property, both public and private, disappears. Today, most citizens feel overwhelmed by their helplessness in the face of this mounting crime on all sides.

A second factor responsible for violence stems from the increasing militance of the hitherto passive, neglected segments of the community. In the past the residents of central city and the other ghetto areas accepted their fate with a passive-aggressive acquiescence. Now they are demanding to be heard. Demonstrations and confrontations are on the increase. When these do not bring change fast enough, riots, arson, bombing and other forms of violent behavior develop. Violence occurs when other techniques to cope with stressful situations have failed. The history of the United States indicates that violence has always been acceptable behavior. The mass media, newspapers, magazines, movies and television stress violence. In fact, they foster a culture of violence.

In such a setting, the mutual distrust between the dominant group and those who feel discriminated against, sets the stage for potential violent outbreak. Ghettos are filled with frustration and despair as the thousands living there find themselves ill-prepared to function in the existing system. Many are products of broken homes, with limited education and lack of work skills. Feeling alienated, unloved, and unwanted, they vent their anger against the world around them. The police, as symbols of the repressive community, become targets for assault. In turn this may arouse militancy in some law officers. The taxpaying citizenry, alarmed by the attacks on them and their institutions, become increasingly hostile. A new phenomenon is the development of paramilitary and vigilante groups seeking to physically control the violence emanating from the ghetto.

Not only the ghetto dweller acts out against society. Today children from affluent, middle-class homes become involved in vandalism, theft, drug abuse and other antisocial behavior. Too often they come from families who show inconsistency in their values or the love for their children. Where gifts and money take the place of love and emotional interaction, children do not acquire a sense of identity or purpose. They act out their frustrations in violence, alcohol or drug abuse, or sexual delinquency.

Some drop out of school or out of work. Others may seek escape from the urban life and its dissatisfactions in the seeming freedom of communal living.

It is a sad fact that violence in the cities seems destined to increase. The National Advisory Commission on Civil Disorders report indicates that whatever choices are made to resolve the ghetto problem, friction and violence to a greater or lesser extent is inevitable.[8] A continuation of our present pattern means polarization and the permanent establishment of two societies; one predominantly white, located in the suburbs, in smaller cities, and in outlying areas, and one largely black, located in central cities. This will result in sustained violence in the cities. The timing, scale, nature, and repercussions of such violence cannot be foreseen.

An alternative, called the *enrichment choice*, is designed to improve the quality of life in the ghetto. This calls for massive expenditures of tax money. Even if adopted, such a program would give rise to undue expectations in ghetto residents beyond the capabilities of prompt delivery. This would be followed by frustration, despair and violent reaction against society. Only over many years can such a program reduce the level and frequency of urban disorder.

A third alternative, called the *integration choice*, would permit the underprivileged to leave the ghetto of the central city to live anywhere in the city or its suburbs. This means providing low-cost housing close to work opportunities. Schools would be integrated to provide quality education to all children. In the commission's report, only this choice offers the possibility of reversing the profoundly divisive trend so evident in the metropolitan areas. However, it is threatening to a large segment of the white population who are prepared to resist any such change, by violence if necessary.

The City Today

In his book *Future Shock*, Alvin Toffler discusses the accelerating changes underway in our lives and in the world.[9] Change is taking place so fast that it is producing psycho-biologic disorders due to man's inability to adapt. The cities show even less adaptability in the face of swift social and technological change. Historically the cities developed in a crazy patchwork without planning and have become functionally unsuited for the pressures of today. While cities came into existence to serve people, they have lost sight of this purpose. The building of high-rises or expressways has become increasingly important with thought given neither to their aesthetic effects nor to their effect on the lives of the urban dwellers. Not only is the city unable to provide physical security for its citizenry, it cannot provide adequate health services for the poor, the uninformed, or the undemanding. Medical and social services suffer from fragmentation, limited personnel and poor distribution. As cities have lost their sense of unity, purpose, and identity, there has been an accompanying social disorganization. There is little long-range planning; most energies are directed to responding to crisis situations.

Originally the city offered man a sense of community with his fellows. Today, such a sense of community rarely exists. Concerned about himself, his family and his employment, the average citizen has little motivation to become involved. There is less interest in helping his neighbor. Man finds himself living isolated in a city that does not seem to care about him. Too often his job has become repetitively monotonous, giving him no sense of personal involvement or accomplishment. His child is exposed to a school system which is breaking down under the many demands made on it and which too often provides inadequate education. The average citizen feels trapped by circumstances beyond his control, as he finds his everyday life a seemingly endless stream of bad news, crises, and confrontations. The jails and detention centers filled to overflowing with adults and youth are symbols of failure to adapt in an increasingly complex environment. Prison riots have become the response to their inhumanity and dehumanization.

Prospects for the Future

The history of mankind is recorded in the rise and demise of cities. Most urbanologists predict the death of cities as we know them unless drastic changes come about very soon. The city must recapture what Mumford called its *life-nurturing* function to better meet the needs of its residents.[10] The individual must have some involvement in decision making; in particular the underprivileged must have some voice at the decision making level. Help must be provided for those not fitting into city life. This means finding jobs for the unskilled, providing better housing, recreation, medical and social services.

We are all interdependent; when a city loses its sense of identity and purpose everyone is hurt. The problem of the ghetto involves everyone. An epidemic in the ghetto does not stay within the ghetto but can run rampant through the city. The breakdown in family life in the slums results in youngsters who grow up to be social problems to the entire community. Good health for the community, both physical and psychological, is indivisible. Programs must be instituted to provide assistance to families under stress before they disintegrate. This includes crisis centers, counselling and treatment programs.

The community must become more supportive of the educational system, even if this requires increased expenditures of money. Without the necessary education, children will not be prepared for their roles as adults in a fast-changing world. Education must be geared to preparation for coping with an increasingly complex world. Youth must be provided better alternatives than now exist. This means honest guidelines to help them understand their biological, sexual, and psychological entities. They need a chance to grow at their own pace with relative freedom from the pressures and anxieties of the adult world. They must be permitted to have a meaningful involvement in the affairs of the city, otherwise their energies will too often find an outlet in destructive, antisocial behavior.

Both the young and the poor are demanding a happier future. Through television and observing life around them, they realize that the material rewards of the affluent society are being denied them. There is less acceptance of gradualism and more demand for instant gratification. Feelings of being shut out generate protest marches, confrontation and open conflict. Enfranchisement and increasing political involvement are but the first steps to bringing the young and the poor to a bargaining position where they can influence those events that affect their lives. Conflict is reduced when these hitherto powerless groups achieve the strengths necessary for negotiation and meaningful discussion with the power structure of the city.

Can our knowledge of human interaction based on psychiatric, psychological and sociological experience, contribute to the restoration of our crumbling cities? One such experiment is underway in Lawrence, Kansas.[11] This community has in recent years experienced open conflict between blacks and whites, arson, student violence and death. In his book, *Listening to America*, William Moyers said of Lawrence:

> The town is large enough to harbor several communities with their own way of life. It is small enough for every citizen to feel the impact of colliding values. The people I met looked at events through the lens of their own personal experience and defined truth by what they saw. So fiercely had each adherent sworn loyalty to his part of the whole, that the idea of community—of a place where people exist competitively without malice—would be hard to repair.[12]

The Menninger Foundation was invited to assist Lawrence, initially by establishing police-community relations groups. The original project was to improve the police image but it was quickly evident that this was only one facet of a bigger problem. The task was to get all the diverse groups in Lawrence to meet together in good faith to define the real problems of that community. Six months of preparation were required before the workshop groups could begin, due to the suspicion and mistrust present in a sharply divided, polarized city. Once the workshops commenced, people learned how others felt about Lawrence's problems of intolerance, prejudice, insufficient work opportunities, insufficient vocational training, inadequate public transportation, inadequate housing, inadequate compensation for police, firemen and other public employees and the difficulties in the school district.

A member of the white vigilante group, a *crusty conservative*, became chairman of the overall steering committee. As he said, "We were so afraid of each other that we'd forgotten that we're all human beings." Similarly, everyone involved in the workshops began to understand the attitudes, problems, fears, and misapprehensions of his fellow-citizens. Most found their own points of view changed as they saw the situation more clearly.

The initial workshops were held in Topeka because there were no neutral meeting places in Lawrence. With the assistance of the Menninger staff, the workshops were directed to evaluate the city's problems and to develop specific solutions. The workshops produced about 80 suggestions to improve community relations. These included allowing citizens to ride as observers in police cars, continuing the workshop programs, establishing a day care center and increasing the staff in the human relations department. There were recommendations for improved police-community relations, for more involvement in the schools and their problems, for more job opportunities and in particular better relations between blacks and whites.

It is too soon to determine what effect this approach has had on the citizens of Lawrence. The first steps have been taken to rebuild a community hitherto fragmented and at war within itself. Perhaps this will be the direction for the future; using the behavioral sciences we may salvage the cities.

Does City Planning Offer Any Solutions for the Future?

Too much planning has been done at a distance with no real understanding of the needs of the population being served. Rarely are the ghetto residents involved in policy or decision making. In the absence of spokesmen or ombudsmen to voice complaints, their only power is the threat of disruption and violence. Even planning for middle-class housing has demonstrated an unawareness of psychological factors. Recently, a model housing project outside Stockholm opened, reflecting the most advanced thinking in community planning. However, the residents have become embittered and disillusioned to find their new community is sterile, devoid of those amenities, shops, taverns, theaters and parks, where people can congregate and develop personal contacts. Brasilia is another city where the emphasis was placed on unusually attractive government buildings with minimal consideration given to needs of the residents of the city.

A recent book, *Cities Fit to Live In,* discusses the physical, psychological and political problems of the cities.[13] A number of trends are apparent. Most important, the open city where people can walk about freely is a thing of the past. Urban living is becoming more like that of the medieval period when cities had walls, gates and armed patrols. In the future, theaters, bars and restaurants open for evening business would be grouped in *evening squares* where enough people would be present to discourage crime.[14] Isolated businesses would either close or move into these enclaves. Industrial, commercial and daytime businesses would be located in areas that could be locked at night. Residential areas would be linked by expressways. Obviously such a compartmentalized city would be devoid of any sense of community.

For the individual city-dweller high-rise apartments or residential *compounds* would provide fortified living arrangements. Man would become a troglodyte, cut off from his neighbors. A description of this cave-dwelling life in Chicago's Marina City graphically depicts these trends.[15] The predominate theme is a basic mistrust. Contact with neighbors is avoided. There is an absence of communal meeting places. Guards, electronic gates and television viewers control the entrances. A majority of the 50,000 residents are single but there are few opportunities for meeting each other. The writer, describing his life in Marina City, found that after several weeks he still had no ways of meeting his neighbors. Despite the human need for personal contact, impersonality and distance colors life in the Marina Cities of today and tomorrow.

Crime is a problem that cities must face both today and in the future. Much criminal activity is associated with individuals who, for a variety of reasons, strike out against the social structure. Unchecked, it portends continuing human jungles where crime would be frequent, widespread, and perhaps out of police control, even in the daytime.[16] Subcultures of violence would be localized in areas of even more homogeneous lower-class populations than today. However, organized crime presents even greater problems. Through control of the drug traffic it furthers the victimization of youth. The financial strengths of organized crime permit the corruption of police and law enforcement and increasing influence on government at all levels. Too often it controls city hall. The invasion of legitimate businesses, labor unions, and the stock market give organized crime power, that, unchecked, may permit it to compete with city, state and federal governments.

Doxiadis has attempted to predict the nature of the urban setting in the years ahead. He anticipates that the present world population of three billion people will increase in the 21st century to at least 20 billion and perhaps as many as 50 billion persons. The urban population will be 33 times greater than now, occupying an area 60 to 100 times the size of today's urban developments. Accompanying this will be an even greater number of cars, machines and buildings. The scale of the city will completely dwarf man. It will probably be beyond his comprehension and he will find himself more unable to cope with it. In the absence of city planning, the cities of the future will be more ugly, devoid of parks and the amenities which previously brought pleasure to the citizens and grace and dignity to the cities. Without planning he sees nothing but disaster. It is his belief that this planning offers the best hope for viable cities where man can live comfortably; otherwise city life will become less human and increasingly more intolerable. It is his hope that the seemingly irresistible drive towards self-destruction that colors city life today can be reversed.[17]

Whenever man has realized the possibility of his destruction through natural disasters such as earthquakes, fire, flood or tornado, or through the man-made catastrophes of warfare or rebellion, he has learned to join with his neighbors to cope with the common threat. We must hope that the mounting pressures and threats of destruction of the city and the health of its residents are intimately intertwined. We must recognize that injury to our neighbor can be an injury to us; we can no longer remain detached. We are our brother's keeper.

Seeley has said that either the city becomes civilization's conscience or else it is only a population trap and a behavioral sink.[18] The city must be shaped to one in which the ordinary individual will find the opportunity to express himself in the best possible way as a person and in his work. If we continue to permit the city to grow and develop haphazardly, it will destroy man. We must shape our cities in their physical settings and their social contexts for the people who are going to live in them. Man must feel that he is in control of his community. Whether this can happen before time runs out only the future will tell.

Toynbee still offers some hope for the future. He recently said, "What mankind needs is a new way of life with new aims, new ideals and a new order of priorities. Health and happiness are more valuable than wealth and power. In our heritage from our ancestors we have spiritual treasures on which we can draw for inspiration in trying to shape our future."[19]

BIBLIOGRAPHY

1. Toynbee, A. (Ed.): *Cities of Destiny.* New York, McGraw-Hill, 1967, p. 14.
2. Toynbee: *op. cit.,* p. 27.
3. Welfare Rolls Shrink—Costs Go Up. *San Francisco Examiner,* Nov. 12, 1971.
4. Selye, H.: *The Stress of Life.* New York, McGraw-Hill, 1956.
5. Doxiadis, C. A.: The Coming World City. In Toynbee (Ed.): *op. cit.,* pp. 345-358.
6. Srole, L., Langer, T. S., Michael, S. T. *et al.: Mental Health in the Metropolis: The Midtown Manhattan Study.* New York, McGraw-Hill, 1962.
7. Rogers, M. L., and Blackwell, B.: Personal Communication. May, 1971.
8. *Report of the National Advisory Commission on Civil Disorders.* New York, Dutton, 1968.
9. Toffler, A.: *Future Shock.* New York, Random House, 1970.
10. Mumford, L.: *The City in History.* New York, Harcourt Brace, 1961, p. 575.
11. McMahon, P. A.: Species Endangered: Creating an Acceptable Environment. *Kansas City Star,* Aug. 29, 1971. Reprinted in *Menninger Perspective,* 2(6):25-29, 1971.
12. Moyers, W. D.: *Listening to America.* New York, Harper's Magazine Press, 1971, p. 122.
13. McQuade, W. (Ed.): *Cities Fit to Live In.* New York, Macmillan, 1971.
14. Angel, S.: Discouraging Crime Through City Planning. Working

Paper No. 75, Center for Planning and Development Research, University of California, Berkeley, 1968. In McQuade (Ed.): *op. cit.*, p. 20.

15. Blumhurst, R.: Welcome to Marina City—The Shape of the New Style. In McQuade (Ed.): *op. cit.*, pp. 26-29.

16. Gold, R.: Urban Violence and Contemporary Defensive Cities. In McQuade (Ed.): *op. cit.*, pp. 4-19.

17. Doxiadis: *op. cit.*, p. 348.

18. Seeley, J.: Remaking the Urban Scene: New Youth in an Old Environment. *Daedalus,* 97:1124-1139, 1968.

19. Toynbee, A.: Toynbee on the Next Ten Years. *San Francisco Sunday Chronicle.* Jan. 17, 1971, p. 4.

Chapter 18

SUMMARY OF WORKSHOP PROCEEDINGS

STEVE ALLEN

THANK YOU, Dr. Auerback, for your generous introduction. Since you raised the question as to whether—my parents being vaudevillians—I ever slept in a dresser drawer, the answer is no— we couldn't afford a dresser.

Well, this has been a most stimulating conference. I arrived here three days ago, refreshed and energetic, eager for what was to come. Now, after three days of listening, speaking, taking notes, studying and discussing from early morning till late at night, I am utterly exhausted. In which condition I am called upon to summarize these proceedings.

I am comforted by the knowledge that the very futility of my assignment will merit me your sympathy. In this connection I am reminded of a very funny story. But I shall resist the temptation to tell it.

The title of my address, like that of Mr. Rozenfeld, as rendered in the program is inaccurate. It has no title. In a sense it isn't even an address. It's more an exercise in presumption.

Being an expert on nothing that has been discussed here I am, of course, the most qualified to discuss everything because I am uninhibited by those sharply defined professional boundaries that limit the rest of you.

I might be considered, in this context, a lay expert. No, come to think of it, I'm not even an expert on that. I throw in a bit of vulgarity so that you young people will feel at home.

But, in all conceit, I have a few observations, and questions, about some of the things we have heard during these three stimulating days.

Since the discussions themselves did not, indeed could not have, followed a straight, disciplined line of inquiry, my comments on them then constitute chiefly a catalogue of your modest digressions, to which I may perhaps add one or two of my own.

There were countless endearing indications, during these meet-

ings, of our naive humanity, which it is always particularly refreshing to encounter in an assemblage of sophisticated practitioners of one discipline or another.

For example, even here, despite the fame and importance of a
given speaker, despite the breadth of experience of members of
this audience—and despite the great unlikelihood that the next
person to walk into this room at a given moment might have
been President Nixon, Mao Tse Tung, or the returned Christ—
nevertheless every time someone walked in during an address
almost every head turned away from the speaker and glanced,
however casually, toward the door.

And despite your depth of understanding and compassion,
there were hostile glares directed at those seized by uncon-
trollable fits of coughing, and even at the inanimate device that is
recording these proceedings.

The high-pitched, wavering tone it has emitted this morning
I found first annoying, then nostalgically comforting in that it
reminded me of the sound of the old radiators that heated so
many of the rooms in which I lived as a child.

Dr. Auerback, intending to refer to Sarah Lawrence College,
called it *David* Lawrence, and then, in response to your laughter,
said, "Make of it what you will."

I respectfully suggest, Doctor, that in this professional context
what is made of it will have to be what *you* will.

Dr. Erika Freeman has told us among other interesting things,
that in a sense England was our mother, France was our mistress
and Germany our teacher.

She did not identify our *father*, which would seem to confirm
our present low opinion of ourselves.

Her point that we ought to judge ideas on their own merits
rather than solely in regard to their source is precisely that which
led to the development of a new game (for which I served as
consultant) called *Strange Bedfellows,* one of a series designed to
teach all of us how to think.

Dr. Tietz's reference to asterisks and the numerous and lengthy
footnotes in his paper reminded me of an insight (or at least a
crazy idea) that occurred to me some years ago when I participated in the experimental program on the effects of LSD conducted by Dr. Sydney Cohen at UCLA.

That was at a time, of course, before the abuse of the drug had emerged as a serious social problem.

I envisioned a page of a book, every word of which was followed by an asterisk, with footnotes.

But . . . in the footnotes, too, every word was followed by an asterisk.

In a time when many, particularly among the young, have grown increasingly cynical about the competence and dedication of political figures, it is encouraging to hear from so able and dedicated a public servant as Mr. Lanterman.

I was greatly enlightened by my exposure to Dr. Bierer's theories, impressed by his accomplishments, and charmed by his company.

Dr. Bierer believes that the solution to the mental health problems of our times is much too large and complex a job for psychiatrists and the mental health people alone. Dr. Auerback's sobering recital makes the dimensions of the problem alarmingly clear. The collaboration and involvement of a multidisciplinary group of professionals is clearly required. Even if Dr. Bierer were wrong philosophically, he is inescapably right on this point.

But his achievements argue persuasively for the essential validity of his approach, for he has contributed many significant innovations to social psychiatry: day and night hospitals, self-determining and self-governing therapeutic clubs, therapeutic communities, and others. Dr. Bierer believes that mental illness as such does not exist. He also believes—as now apparently every informed person does—that our system of legal justice and punishment is ineffective if not irrational.

One of the more interesting subsidiary questions raised concerns the extent to which the political Right, which has long been active in the field of mental health as the force of the opposition to it, is now making use of Dr. Szsaz and Dr. Bierer as weapons with which to attack psychiatry and the mental health movement generally. There are a number of historical factors involved in this rightist paranoia: (1) Anti-Semitism, because many psychiatrists are Jews, (2) the Church-versus-Freud, and (3) the suspiciousness characteristic of political fanaticism. Those who *need* treatment but deny the need are pleased to hear Dr. Bierer say, "There's no such thing as mental illness," because it confirms their sense of righteousness.

I am not referring to responsible conservatives here but to the traditional force of know-nothing reaction.

The large question Dr. Bierer raises, being complex, is still unresolved. In recent years, as you know, there has been a return to emphasis, in some quarters, upon *physical* factors related to mental illness, if Dr. Bierer will pardon the expression.

That kind of genetic chromosomal abnormality, for example, which has a correlation with antisocial criminal behavior would be a case in point. There are studies, too, as you are aware, of differences in blood chemistry between those who are schizophrenics and those who are not. And there are the obvious questions presented by the successful results obtained by the administration of such drugs as *lithium* in modifying human behavior for the better.

It was only recently, historically speaking, that we discovered that separate parts of the brain governed separate bodily functions, muscular movements, speech, sight, memory, and so forth. But uncharted horizons now beckon in that specific area of the brain out of which the *emotions* arise.

I suspect little is known, too, about such refined areas of specialization as the *mathematical* or *musical* functions. If the strict environmentalists present will forgive me, it has always seemed to me preposterous to assert that if a genius can compose a symphony and play the piano brilliantly at the age of six, the fact is explained purely by the availability of a better-than-adequate music teacher.

I know from personal experience that the gift of musical composition has nothing whatever to do with being taught. The mechanical components of the art can be taught but the essential gift, the ability to synthesize factors in previously unimagined ways is just that—if one posits a giver—a gift, a puzzling accident, difficult to explain even in terms of standard Darwinian theory, since it hardly is necessary to the survival of the species.

In a book written some years ago I advanced the hypothesis that the gift of religious spirituality, which is clearly more pronounced in some individuals than others, may have its focus literally in brain tissue. I hasten to add that since the firm belief that God made all things logically requires the belief that He created the human brain, the theory is in no way incompatible with religious philosophy generally.

It is interesting that some years later, when we began to receive reports, most of them scholarly and some of them from Dr. Bierer, attesting to either the reality or illusion of religious and spiritual insights under the influence of LSD and similar drugs, I began to feel that my theory was given substantial support in the form of consistent if by no means conclusive evidence.

Dr. Branch's presentation had the appeal we always sense in those arguments that conform with our own prejudices. I was especially intrigued by his reminding us of the importance of the emotional attitude of the therapist in relating to the patient, as dramatized in the story of the practitioner who reported that on five particular days his patients seemed especially cheerful and open. As you will recall, these were the days on which he had taken benzedrine.

This is consistent with my own experience in being frequently interviewed over a period of years, in connection with my television activities. I noticed early that the interviewers who were themselves extroverts tended to describe me as lively, witty and genial, whereas those who were more introverted tended to describe me as shy, withdrawn, uncommunicative, etc.

There were a thousand-and-one tempting digressions, the following out of which could take literally many lifetimes. For example, Dr. Kennedy referred to *glossalalia*, the speaking in strange tongues.

I would like to know if tape-recordings of the phenomenon have been made, if written transcripts of these recordings have been rendered, and if both have been subjected to analysis by disinterested linguistic scholars.

Dr. Kennedy's remarks struck a particularly responsive emotional chord.

One could not fail to be impressed by his enthusiasm for the campaign to, as he put it, *unscrew the pew*.

He expressed the idea with such force, in fact, that I would not be surprised to see him shortly dispense with the negative prefix.

But the relevance of the self-treating encounter group to the essential work of the church is clear. Just as Christians civilized the savage tribes of Europe, so the humanist tradition has worked tirelessly for centuries to civilize Christians. It is encouraging to observe that its influence continues unabated.

One of the most touching illustrations drawn by Dr. Kennedy concerned the man who was unable to weep at recollection of his own misfortunes but did so when one of the women in the group told him she loved him for his sympathetic response to her own recital.

The tears that flow in response to love are more mysterious than those that help relieve the sense of tragedy. I find that I am moved to tears at the spectacle of the reconciliation of enemies. There is a sudden rush of feeling that comes from the appreciation of the beautiful aspects of human communication.

I found Dr. Brill's presentation of particular interest, although perhaps at our next convocation we might be privileged to see a slide projection of that mysterious picture of him with the two Yugoslavian girls.

His description of the alienation of American youth was most complete and detailed. One must, it seems to me, agree with his conclusion that the state of consciousness of today's young people is different in kind, as well as in degree, compared to the youth of earlier generations.

One reason may be that today's technology, TV, radio, films, magazines, video-tape and audio equipment, brings our social reality into focus to a degree unprecedented in all history. And, in today's world, to become *aware* is to become *angry*.

One may become angry at the social injustice suffered by others or by oneself.

But it is remarkable how many ancient beliefs are currently relevant and popular among young people. As regards the materialistic biases of our generation, what are the young saying but that the love of money is the root of a great deal of evil?

In saying that they want to *enjoy* their work, not just perform it for money, the young are repeating the medieval theologians, are they not?

Unfortunately we resort to the specious as well as to what has been valid from the storehouse of history. Frank Kelly calls ours *The Age of Paranoia.* Who would have supposed it would follow the Age of Reason? And who would have predicted, in a period of spectacular scientific achievement, that the superstition of the Dark Ages, belief in witchcraft, astrology, fortune-telling, and diabolism would culminate in today's very similar wave of occultism and deliberate rejection of rational standards?

To the extent that the young regard the rest of us as enemies it might be argued that their position is most fortunate. For example, if you could tell the Marxists of the world that all capitalists will be dead in another 20 or 30 years, their joy would know no bounds. If you could assure the west that all communists would shortly vanish from our planet they, too, would be pleased. Well, the young can literally be assured that all of the older generation will be gone before long, after which the young will perceive that their most formidable adversaries are their own age.

And soon, all those who have said "Don't listen to anybody over 30" will be over 30 themselves, and presumably without an audience.

As for the rebelliousness of today's youth, many of you must be tempted to hope that some magical method might be found whereby it could be stamped out. Not only is the hope utterly incapable of realization but, even if the thing were possible, it ought never to be done, for by inhibiting the rebellious instinct we would be running counter to one of mankind's most fundamental drives: the need to identify what is wrong in his physical context, to oppose what he regards as contemptible, and to construct a better social order. I naturally do not suggest that every fourteen-year-old who breaks a window consciously articulates such a philosophy, but rebellious acts as a class grow out of such a need and are consistent with such a philosophy. The rebel without a cause, as the brilliant Robert Lindner suggested, is dangerous. But the rebel with a good cause will be our salvation.

Both Dr. Brill and Dr. Girvetz commented on the problem of violence in today's youth culture. In my view, the underlying danger of violence, above and beyond the ovbious physical destruction it causes: the deaths, the maimings, the personal tragedy, is that when it becomes institutionalized and apparently legitimized by philosophers or other spokesmen it unleashes dark, dangerous, poorly-understood forces in the human heart, forces that may leap out and eventually consume those who called them forth.

In World War II we observed the atrocities committed by Germans and Japanese, while ignoring those perpetrated by ourselves and our allies. But the evildoers seemed more than evil in our eyes. All men, after all, are partly evil. Our enemy seemed monstrous. Clearly there were psychopaths, sadistic bullies and other such wearing German uniforms. But I think most atrocities are committed by very average people, when they have been programmed to kill and absolved of guilt before the fact. The My Lai murders are a case in point.

I recall, in this connection, a young man who appeared several years ago as a guest on one of my television programs. He had been captured by the Viet Cong while fighting in Vietnam and had been a prisoner for, as I recall, a year or so. Eventually he escaped and made his way back to safety.

When the program was over on the evening that he appeared, I invited him to join our production staff for our customary dinner in a restaurant near our theatre in New York. I emphasize that this young man was very personable. He was, in a sense, the All-American boy. Not remarkably superior or inferior, he had a simple, rural, small-town America manner about him. I would be very surprised to learn that he ever had suffered emotional problems of any sort. Nevertheless while we were discussing the war with him, in answer to my question as to what he thought the ultimate solution might be, he said, "I think we ought to drop the bomb on the Chinese."

"You mean," I said, "attack China's military installations?"

"No," he said, "we ought just to wipe 'em all out."

"With hydrogen bombs?"

"Right."

"You mean," I said, "kill six or seven hundred million mostly civilian men, women and children?"

"I know it sounds terrible," he said, "and it *would* be terrible.

But, the way I look at it, we're going to have to fight them in the long run anyway. Better them than us."

So here we see an instance of a perfectly normal and I suppose essentially decent young fellow evidencing a moral insensitivity that is basically the sort that made the Nazis and more militant Japanese of World War II seem so monstrously evil from our point of view.

Dr. Girvetz's delineation of the problem of violence in our culture clearly suggested that it is on the increase and side-by-side with the common view that today there is a greater incidence of mental and emotional disturbance in our society than at any time in our history; it is remarkable that Dr. Bierer's theories relating to doing away with mental hospitals and prisons are being advanced at a time when one might otherwise assume that they would be building *more* hospitals and prisons.

Another vitally important question, suggested by Mr. Kelly, is: in a presumably *representative* society, who really represents the people? It is not today the easiest question in the world to answer.

Part of the problem is that running for any political office is an incredibly expensive undertaking. Running for high office takes millions of dollars. The sources from which such funds are donated understandably enough expect some sort of return on their investment.

But in response to the growing awareness of this dilemma, there are signs of emerging programs designed to alleviate the distress. Ralph Nader and his organizations are a result of the feeling of helplessness on the part of the average citizen. *Common Cause* is another. So is the *consumer revolution* generally. Ombudsman experiments are springing up. Environmental conservationists are making their influence felt. Radio and TV stations are not only editorializing but are offering free time to spokesmen of points-of-view differing with those of station management.

I take these as hopeful indications.

At least two of our speakers, Mr. Rozenfeld and Dr. Cobbs, emphasized the destructive effects of inadequate social environments upon those forced to live in them. In the physical sense it has long been obvious that poverty and squalor lead to greater incidence of disease and a higher death rate. But only relatively recently have we learned of the harm that poverty does to the mind and the spirit.

Is it possible, however, that the harm is done in a secondary rather than direct sense, in that the conditions of the urban ghetto, as well as of rural poverty, tend to destroy the family, then bring the collapse of adequate parent-child relationships that directly cripples many children psychologically?

It is fascinating to observe to what extent the psychologically destructive potential of many of our unpleasant social problems is now being emphasized.

We have long known that litter, garbage, and sewerage are unedifying to observe, but we are now being told that they also contribute to our societal *neuroses.*

Perhaps one solution, in the context of our free-enterprise biases, would be to find a way to make sewerage and garbage commercially valuable. Then it would be responsibly handled.

Concerning racial confrontation, I found Dr. Cobbs' remarks of very great interest and I plan to read his book *Black Rage.*

In introducing him Dr. Brill observed that although over a million copies of his book had been sold, Dr. Cobbs reported receiving *very little money*, a fact which by itself would make his rage understandable.

One was pleased to hear his recommendation of the Jeffersonian approach to oppression. Almost everyone is opposed to some form of tyranny, but few seem to regard *all* forms as intolerable. Perhaps because most of our forefathers fled from oppression to these shores Americans have long been opposed to all oppression except that which we perpetrated ourselves. But our foreign policy dilemma at present hangs on precisely the question as to how one should oppose oppression. Do we oppose it only within our national borders? If not, how do we respond to the pleas of the oppressed in other parts of the world? Neither of the two large alternatives is entirely satisfactory; consequently we grieve and are uncertain.

Small, revealing things hold a special sort of interest, whether we observe them in the behavior of individuals or groups. I noticed, for example, that the applause for Dr. Cobbs reached a higher volume of intensity than that received by any of the *white* speakers at this conference.

This is consistent with my hypothesis that in the entertainment field, all conditions being generally equal, black performers will usually receive somewhat more applause from *white* audiences than will white entertainers.

The facile explanation is obviously: white guilt. But perhaps something more is involved. Perhaps such applause is one of the few gestures of goodwill that whites know how to make towards blacks. It isn't much, but it *is* something.

One of the most fascinating exchanges—as Dr. Freeman has reminded us—came when Dr. Cobbs characterized Dr. Park's concept of the ghettoization of prison populations as *shoddy.*

We do not have time here to take up the details of the controversy itself, but we might learn something from the nature of Dr. Park's response to Dr. Cobb's verbal attack. *Your* response was not to gasp but to *smile.* Several of you, in fact, turned to *me* and smiled, as if to say, "Get a load of what's going on." I did.

But Dr. Park's response was primarily emotional, perhaps visceral, as evidenced by the immediate breakdown in his sentence-structure. As the tape-recorded transcript will show, he communicated in various unconnected fragments of sentences for a few seconds and then counterattacked, not ad hominem but ad civita. What else might one expect, it occurred to Dr. Park to ask, from someone who lived in San Francisco?

It is certainly not my purpose here either to make light of Dr. Park or to force him to relive those few awkward moments during which egos were wounded and exposed.

My intention is rather to emphasize the frailty of our capacity for reason. Passion may occasionally inspire men to eloquence but it is more likely to render them less rather than more articulate and reasonable. Dr. Park then, stands for everyman. Perhaps none of us are truly graceful under surprise attack.

I was myself subjected to critical aspersions and had my loyalty questioned by a woman in the audience I addressed here locally on Friday at noon.

My response, too, was to feel a surge of emotion. It was low level but its components were recognizable as fear and anger.

So we all carry this ancient animal burden, part protection and part curse. The knowledge should make us more charitable in dealing with those with whom we disagree.

Dr. Girvetz has become a typical figure in the contemporary American political drama, the liberal who, though he does not substantially change himself, feels the ground shift under him, as a result of which social earthquake he comes to rest at a point farther to the right on the political spectrum than he is accustomed to.

Today's liberal is historically symptomatic, however, in a sense that merits him far better treatment than the casual dismissal or outright contempt he sometimes receives from those to his left or those who feel that he has not done enough for them. For the values and institutions the liberal defends are those that were unknown for countless ages, those that were prayed for, dreamed for, struggled for, died for by a now-faceless mass of valiant souls who suffered under a thousand tyrannies and longed pathetically for the freedom to speak their minds, to write or otherwise disseminate their views, to travel without harsh restriction, to worship or not, as it pleased them, to congregate with others at will, to live in such social conditions that one could at least *pursue* happiness, insure domestic tranquility, and function as both reason and passion have told the best among us down through the ages man was meant to function.

The crimes of the Industrial Revolution rudely cut across these libertarian dreams. Clearly the people deserved a large measure of economic security. It is perhaps the primary task of this century to determine if the inherent contradiction between *freedom* on the one hand and *security* on the other can be reasonably balanced.

Even now the liberal stands between the Radical Left and the Radical Right, who might today be at each other's throats if it were not for his intervention.

The liberal is as open to criticism as everyone else, but in concentrating on his shortcomings we must not lose sight of the herculean achievements of progressive forces over the centuries in advancing human freedom.

Speaking of freedom, a gentleman in the audience expressed a combination of horror and surprise that a recent survey shows that young children voted *against* our constitutional guarantees of liberty, against free speech, against legal rights, and so forth.

But I would have thought that children were recognized as notoriously intolerant. They are trained to *receive* love rather than to give it, to receive material necessities rather than to provide them to others. An infant is a squalling, screaming bundle of insistent demands, not a beneficent dispenser of blessings and concern for others.

Faced with the question as to how to deal with evil-doers, children almost invariably recommend harsh punishment because they are motivated by their horror of the evil done, not by those sophisticated and tolerant standards which it took adult mankind untold hundreds of thousands of years to develop, and which even now are shakily buttressed by popular sentiment even in the most civilized societies.

Because of their exposure to TV and films, children incline to believe that the way to treat a bad man is to have Gary Cooper or John Wayne or Jack Webb shoot him on the spot. And they are not alone.

Dr. Bierer wisely draws our attention to the fact that on the one hand we have millions of wealthy or retired people who report that they have little to do to productively occupy their time, while on the other hand almost all necessary social agencies report a shortage of helpful workers. Clearly the idle personnel must somehow be directed toward the areas of need. Perhaps experienced management people, given the opportunity for public communication, could productively deal with this problem.

Something along this line is already being done by the *Thiokol Chemical Corporation,* for whom I recently narrated a documentary film telling of their very positive and productive pro-

gram for training hard-core, unemployable young ghetto people, not only for regular jobs or further academic studies, but,
perhaps most significantly, training them to do the same work by
which they were helped so that they in turn can have a positive,
productive feedback in their ghetto communities. This program
deserves far more public attention than it has received and I recommend it to your further study.

I am troubled by a certain looseness of language which seems
to me symptomatic of our time. In discussing *violence* yesterday
one gentleman said "rats are violent." Others make the claim
that poverty itself is violence upon the poor. Having lived with
both poverty and with rats in my own youth, I know their ugliness.
It is disgusting and disgraceful that men should have to live in
rat-infested tenements. But to bend the word *violence* to cover
this painful-enough reality, it seems to me, confuses rather than
clarifies the issue.

In the debate on obscenity one hears it said that *war* is obscene, that *violence* is obscene. Words are imprecise enough to
begin with, judged as scientific instruments, without our rendering them even more rubbery.

Lastly we were moved by Judge Lodge's recitation of his experience in visiting Atascadero State Hospital and finding that
he was the only judge, out of over 500, who had accepted the inmates' invitation to attend a conference there.

Perhaps there is some connection between Judge Lodge's social conscience and his youth. Such men serve for me as yard-
sticks by which I measure my own passage through time. Partly
I suppose because my health is still good I do not feel as old as I
am, which is 49. But since I reached the middle thirties I began
to notice the strange phenomenon that policemen were starting
to look like high-school boys. Eventually clergymen, doctors, and
now even judges look like college youths.

In closing, I take it that we would agree that there is no one
magic answer, no one philosophical framework within which
all problems will be resolved and all difficulties surmounted.
Those abstractions, representing concrete enough realities, which
elicit hope in our hearts, *education, religion, democracy, free-*

dom, psychiatry, political constitutionalism, even such attractive ideals are not panaceas.

Perhaps I should mention that I am a Christian so that you will understand my fundamental bias in regard to this question. I stand, in other words, among those who hold that religion in essence is a positive force and one capable of influencing human behavior in acceptable directions. But the fact remains that the pages of religious history are stained with such rivers and seas of human blood, that the record of religious practice is blackened by instances of such massive intolerance and fanaticism, that it cannot possibly be responsibly argued that religion pure and simple is *the* answer our hearts seek.

Nor can *education* be that answer. Germany in the 1930's was the best educated nation in Europe. The German people were also highly religious, for that matter; at least they were affiliated with the various Christian churches. But this religious and well-educated people nevertheless perpetrated the horrors, under Hitler's guidance, that led to the massive destruction of World War II.

As for *freedom,* we feel its lack sensitively and its loss even more painfully. Obviously it is a good. But it frequently provides operative room in which countless moral atrocities and obscenities are committed.

It is not a proper response to such understanding to turn *against* education, religion or freedom; we are merely advised against investing overly large amounts of hope in such conditions.

It is perhaps a wonder, or a tribute to our resourcefulness and resiliency, that we know any happiness or intellectual satisfaction at all, given that our existence is quite literally bounded by mystery and death.

Consider the two fundamental concepts by which we locate ourselves, *space* and *time.* Concerning each there are two possible positions, both of which are absurd. Either time began, which is preposterous, since we can easily think of a continuum *before* it began, or it did *not* begin, which we can not think of at all. Either it will end or it will not, both of which are obviously impossible.

As for space, either it is infinite, which can not be the case, or it ends somewhere, which is equally preposterous.

We are born ignorant animals and we die in pain and confusion. In between we can perceive and create things of beauty and value, but part of our tragedy is that they can all be turned to evil ends. Whether we speak of freedom, democracy, education, religion, courage, love, sex; everything that we need to sustain us can also kill us, everything can be abused, as well as used.

This association merits great credit for its attempts to induce man to make the wisest possible use of his mental, spiritual and material resources.

PART VI
EXPERIENTIAL THERAPY

Chapter 19

ART THERAPY

URSULA MAHLENDORF, Ph.D.

A FRIEND RECENTLY REMARKED that in our therapy patients usually did not lose their creativity but rather gained or re-
gained it. Menninger, in his *Vital Balance*,[1] holds out the hope
for people afflicted with mental illness (and for their families),
that such an illness often leads to the stage of *better than well,*
that is to say, to an increase in self-understanding, maturity and
heightened creative achievement. He gives this observation as an
assertion and does not describe the way in which such heightened creativity is reached, just as if this creativity were a by-
product of *getting well.*

Perhaps by describing the process of a gain in creativity, we
can learn something about a therapy successful beyond the mere
alleviation of symptoms. In addition, such a description will serve
to demonstrate the relationship between therapy and art, and to
clarify the ways in which human creativity is freed and nur-
tured at any time in human life.

We all know that children, in their play, show an inventiveness
that later is stifled. In fact, we deplore that our schools neglect
to nurture creativity in our children. We see children's art shows
inspired by a particularly interested teacher and we marvel at
the talent displayed. We read children's stories and we are amazed
at the keenness of observation the child expresses. Despite technical defects, there is a freshness about such work, a directness
of expression, that gives truth and conviction to their paintings
and stories. Except in a few cases, this ability to express oneself
unambiguously, and forthrightly, dies—either slowly or with a
blow.

I remember an afternoon in a boarding school when I was fourteen. I was copying the portrait of a then famous flyer whose
face I liked. I felt I had achieved a fine representation of the
strength of that face, and pleased, showed the drawing to my

311

roommates. I glowed at their approval. I then went to our drawing teacher. She told me that I could produce even a better likeness if I used a system of lines across the page and defined the areas of the face more closely, proceeding to impose these lines on my drawing, redoing some of my lines, erasing others. As the face changed, my drawing was obliterated; what I had thought important, my impression of the face, disappeared.

At the time I did not know what was happening. I felt angry but could not express it; I felt that the teacher did mean to help. I was not strong enough, and no child or beginner is, to defend my vision against an expert—or adult—who is supposed to know what drawing is all about. A more observant teacher and one respectful of the child's vision, might have suggested improvements to be made, might have done another drawing without destroying mine. In any case, I did not draw another line after that afternoon.

The reader might think, so fine, so good, then I did not have enough talent to start with. Many are called, few are chosen. We generally suppose that such deaths need to happen. Who does not know that many patients during some phase of their most intense treatment experience a regression to childhood, usually during hospitalization, and suddenly take to self-expression in whatever occupational therapy is offered; and who has not observed that such attempts at drawing, modelling or any other creative endeavor usually stop as soon as the patient copes better with the situations of his real life in the world.

Such creative expression is a passing phase. Then, too, who has not noted some former promising poets or painters who, in the course of therapy, lost whatever talent they had earlier. Being better adjusted to their living situation, suffering less tension, being more comfortable with themselves, they no longer needed to express themselves through an artistic medium, or so reports go. And what friend of such artists-to-be has not regretted this loss with all awareness of their friends' greater ability to function in their family and community.

The loss of childhood creativity has been pointed out by writers of such different persuasions as Schiller *(Letters on the Aesthetic Education of Mankind)*, Nietzsche *(Zarathustra)* and

Marcuse *(Eros and Civilization).* In different formulations, all three blame this loss on training toward specialization that society exacts from man. For if creativity means freedom, playfulness, spontaneity, naiveté toward tradition, sensuousness, total involvement in a nonutilitarian task, then all creative undertakings must be suspect to a social order that demands of its members conformity to established norms, reliance upon tradition to build upon, specialization in one task that has a useful goal and a sufficient income.

To ensure such results, it is safest to follow certain routines and established traditions (and routines need to be followed also for the sake of stability). We all know that the great artists have not done so, that their achievement has been precisely contrary to the tastes, routines, and goals of their immediate historical periods. And we imagine that their talent must have been so strong that it overcame the temptation toward immediate success. We believe that some unusual kind of madness (Lombroso's *Genius and Madness*) made them persevere at their chosen tasks despite lack of recognition, success and all that goes with it.

The critics of civilization, Schiller (1797), Nietzsche (1884-86), and Marcuse (1957), point out that modern civilization with its affluence no longer needs to exact from man the total sacrifice of emotional and sensuous needs for the sake of success or survival. They assert that other satisfactions than material ones (that are so shortlived and that chain man to ever new and less fulfilling goals) might bring greater fulfillment to man. All three suggest creative expression in the arts as a cure for man's spiritual and emotional ills. It is striking that these recommendations have occupied thinkers for the last two hundred years and that they have found so little acceptance in the civilization to which they were addressed.

The promise of greater happiness was not accepted—why? Ironically, it came into disrepute through the greatest liberating force of the early twentieth century, through Freud. His belief, expressed in *Civilization and Its Discontents,* that some instinctual gratifications must be sublimated into higher forms of expression, artistic, intellectual, or social achievements, led to some startling reaffirmations of earlier prejudices against the artist and

the role of art in culture. For some of his followers, artistic creation became synonymous with regression to and subsequent sublimation of erotic and ambitious unfulfilled wishes. Once man
learned to gratify some of these wishes realistically, he would
no longer need to indulge in symbolic wish fulfillment. For only
the unhappy person has fantasies and "if fantasies become over-
luxuriant and overpowerful, the necessary conditions for an
outbreak of neurosis or psychosis are constituted. . . . A broad
bypath here branches off into pathology."[2]

With this statement of Freud's the old *madness and artist* theory reappeared in a new guise. Hence for some schools of psychiatry the giving up of artistic attempts by the patient signals the
end of regression, the resignation of infantile instinctual demands,
and the realistic adjustment of needs to the environment. For
this reason, there is no longer any need to transform wishes into
expression in paint, words and clay. Artists and art lovers have
rebelled against such an interpretation of art and its role in life.

Another misconception, allied to the first, also derived from
Freud's formulations. In this case, the artist is seen more positively. His ability to transform his instinctual needs, the *achievement* of sublimation, is stressed. And this seems to have been
Freud's own favored interpretation. Such sublimation occa-
sioned suffering, sacrifice. And art was not, as Schiller or Nietzsche claimed, enjoyment, rather it was suffering, the lonely,
misunderstood artist, martyr of Romanticism, made his reap-
pearance with a vengeance. The belief that the artist needed to
suffer, to deny himself instinctual gratification is most curiously
illustrated by the case of the poet Rilke.

In 1912 Rilke, in a depression which threatened his sanity,
turned to his former mistress Lou Andreas Salomé, at the time
studying with Freud at Vienna. He asked her to recommend a
psychiatrist to help him. Lou considered some students of Freud's
whom the poet might consult, but then reconsidered. On the day
before the poet went to see the recommended physician, he received a wire with the recommendation not to undergo treatment. The letter following the telegram reaffirmed Rilke's belief that his emotional suffering was needed to make him into the
great poet he wished to be.

After he had written the *Elegies* and the *Sonnets to Orpheus,* Lou wrote him that this sacrifice of personal comfort to art made possible these achievements, that it had been a "triumph without measure." (I find these words cruel without measure.) Would Rilke have ceased writing had he had psychiatric help? Possibly, if such treatment had been oriented toward the above mentioned first approach to art. It comes as no surprise that Jungian analysis with its stress on art as fulfillment, its lesser fear of regression and its tolerance for deviation from social norms, has had more success with the treatment of artists, the case of Hermann Hesse comes to mind.[3]

Be that as it may, heroic suffering or unbalanced and unhappy compulsion, the curious fact remains that artists of all ages have gone on creating their works against all odds. The more verbal ones among them have insisted that precisely in the process of creating, they felt the most fulfilled and most in touch with themselves and the world. And such happiness, if we are to believe our artists, was not the result of a Pollyannaish denial of the unhappiness, the grief, the regret, the anger, the frustration, the tragedies that we are heir to. Rather their work was an affirmation of the reality and the power of emotions denied by the *well-adjusted* optimist.

What then about the use of creative endeavor in therapy? What aside from assertions about its usefulness, effects, or the promised end product, the *better than well person* of the beginning of our essay? What is the way? Let me first state that such therapy is not a gimmick to be learned in five easy lessons and let me also say that it is not a matter of aesthetic value, achievement, suffering or the like pretensions. For the sake of clarity and conviction let me speak of my experience.

I had consulted Dr. C. four years earlier after an unsuccessful suicide attempt. At the time I thought that I had tried to take my life because I was desperately lonely and overworked. After a few sessions I stopped seeing Dr. C. as I received recognition for my work and resumed a former love relationship. A few weeks later my mother came to visit me from Europe and stayed on with me. In the beginning my mother's staying with me gave me a reason for living, but gradually the strain of having to be total provider and companion for her became too much. Working as a teacher was an almost intolerable burden, sleep without drinking impossible and writing, my favorite occupation till then, a meaningless chore. I did not want to live and I knew that I needed help to be able to live.

In weekly sessions during the next two years, I learned to talk about myself. This was difficult learning since I had not talked about myself ever since early adolescence. That is to say, at about age fifteen I gave up mentioning facts relating to myself. Talking about emotions stopped much earlier, if it was ever encouraged. I remember that at age eight I ceased speaking of aesthetic experiences to my family since they ridiculed them. Nevertheless, precisely such feelings occupied me much of the time as an adolescent and adult.

In order to appear *normal,* I learned to construct a likely childhood story for my later friends. I called it rather cynically to myself "the myth of the happy childhood." I saw to it that the friends I associated with were students of literature and art and hence would not object to an aesthetic or intellectual mode of experience. Learning to speak was learning to feel what I spoke, to *disintellectualize* my experience.

My training in literature, psychology and philosophy at this stage of therapy was a hindrance to emotional understanding rather than a help. I do not think that this needs to be the case. People who have studied these fields with a need to know more deeply and fully will leave themselves open to the emotional understanding of thought and aesthetic form. I studied them as a defense, harshly said as equipment for hiding. A great deal of my deception had also become self-deception. I knew that intellectually, I was to meet it (and I still do) in falsifications of memory, in uncertainty about what I felt. For the most part it seemed to me that during these years I was walking on ice, slippery here, thin there, holding one moment, about to break and breaking the next. Although I trusted my therapist, I was not sure if he would hold me if I fell on or worse, through the ice. I certainly did not know, intellectually or otherwise, what ice meant.

At the end of this period of therapy, I had gained sufficient self-understanding and self-confidence that I realized, on the occasion of my mother's visit to Europe, that I wanted to live my own life. This realization was sudden, as many such *break-throughs* to follow. However, it was prepared slowly by a lessening of tension, by greater confidence in my therapist and greater self-reliance. During this period, participation in a group led by the therapist and in classes in creative stitchery helped me to some extent. The former made me aware of the living problems of others, an awareness from which I had been shut off earlier. The latter provided some occupation other than my usual preoccupation with matters intellectual. Both brought me together with people with whom I had to be honest, even if this honesty consisted in being shy and withdrawn rather than in faking liveliness and in being intellectual as I was earlier.

The extent of my noninvolvement in therapy at that time is amazing to me now. In terms of the emotional energy available to me then (the reliving of old grief, anger and fear, the confusion about who I was and what I felt) I was as involved as I could afford to be.

I resumed therapy after a six months' period in Europe. I lived alone, having left my mother in Germany. At first I was exhilarated by my newly found independence, but I soon became depressed by my actual loneliness and felt guilty about having deserted my mother. In addition some of my old friends reacted to this separation as people do toward a divorce by taking sides with one partner or the other. I attempted to establish new friendships, but being much too shy, withdrawn and preoccupied with my inner confusions, I was unable to establish any sort of meaningful relationship. To drown out loneliness and feeling I drank more heavily than earlier.

On the whole, this entire period which lasted for a year was the most painful and unrewarding one of my therapy, a holding on and waiting, with just sufficient trust in the therapist not to give up. Since I was living in a less stressful situation than earlier, I coped more easily with external problems at work. To the friends I kept, I seemed more at ease, less confused and less withdrawn. To an extent that was true.

"Would you like to take dance therapy?" Dr. C. asked me. I had just been saying that there were times when I felt badly coordinated and not very much at ease with myself. I agreed readily, thinking that a bit more gracefulness and some exercise could do me no harm. A few days later I appeared for my first session in the dance studio. I was tense and apprehensive, afraid of being awkward. The lesson went well and, having taken some modern dance classes earlier, I was fairly proud that I could do almost all the exercises I was asked to do. I left quite happy, having had a good workout. I looked forward to the following session, prepared to move as much as possible to make maximum use of the hour. J., the dance therapist, began to look more and more unhappy during the hour and at its end asked if she could come with me to my session with Dr. C. "Why the hell does she want to use up *my* hour," I thought, but agreed.

We went into Dr. C.'s office and the two began to talk. From amongst the confused noise I heard: "Professorial, knows it all." That obviously referred to me, the rest made no sense. "You know nothing about dancing," Dr. C. said rather sternly, "So why don't you let J. show you." That too made little sense, since I knew I did not know anything about dancing. I did realize though, that I was missing almost everything being done and said, and agreed to let J. "show me," if for no other reason than curiosity.

The next hour J. had me lie down on the floor and close my eyes. I was to feel my body touching the floor, the back of my head, my shoulders, my arms, my back, my buttocks, my thighs, my legs, my heels. Then I was to open my body to the air, to let it touch me all over, let it caress me. As I was lying spread-eagle fashion, J. said all the parts of my body where the air was touching my skin. She then put on a record, and asked me to imagine that the music was flowing over me. Music soon turned into waves; I saw myself at the edge of the ocean; waves were lapping over me, washing me back and forth. I felt like crying.

It seems to me now that it took me a long time to cry, to be angry, to be sad, to be sensuous. I had always *felt like* crying, being angry, or being joyful. I had screened myself from perceiving motion and emotion and regarded the former as merely useful or necessary, the latter as an uncomfortable hindrance at best, a weakness at worst. At first, after an hour of beating in anger on a beat-up bed, of shouting, of moving sensuously, of dancing with exhilaration, I felt rather guilty, even though I thought I had repudiated prudishness.

At other times I felt that I had acted in a rather silly manner, had carried on about *nothing*. Even though we had agreed earlier to throw out intellect and superego during dance, thinking and controlling spontaneity were too much ingrained in me to be simply dismissed; maternal and social injunctions of what was proper behavior and expression of feeling we literally scraped off and wrung out of my body. The immediate gain was that I began to feel alive, to feel myself all there occupying definite space. The language of the body was literal and forthright; if I wanted to escape it, consciously or unconsciously, the therapist at first and later I myself did not let it be silenced.

Often it seemed to me that I was learning a language, a language I had known dimly in early childhood and had forgotten since then. But to learn a language we need a teacher or interpreter. We have to be sure that the teacher will tell us the right words to use, that in a strange country with an alien tongue he will not leave us. Let me illustrate what I mean by such trust, which I had a hard time gaining even in rudimentary form. One day J. asked me to imagine that I was a baby lying in my crib, to feel how I moved my arms and legs. I did so and felt comfortable and warm. J., thinking that I was cold, picked up her coat lying near me. I did not notice that she had done so. As the coat fell over me, I saw something dark fall on me and screamed in terror. Something huge and black, terror, scream, dark, fighting off the smothering with my arms. These were feelings, motions and sensations.

Later I realized the experience was so terrifying because it was totally nonverbal. A second after it all happened, I was halfway back in the present; but for that one moment of terror I lived totally *in* the six months' child's life. I continued crying with fear for a long time, while J. held me and rocked me. I later felt that the two of us had come through a dark whirlpool, and that she had held on to me.

Trust is not gained once and for all in one such experience, but many such experiences help to establish it ever more firmly.

With more confidence in the dance therapist came greater trust in my body, a greater willingness to let it express its needs, its perceptions of itself, its relatedness to others, and its memories. To explore all these possibilities, different groupings proved very helpful. I had dance therapy with J. alone, a mother-daughter or sometimes a sibling interaction; with J. and the therapist, a mother-father-daughter or sometimes a male-female interaction; with a group of women, a sibling interaction.

Let me give examples of explorations of body needs, self-perceptions and the like from dance group sessions. A member of the group states that she still acts in a manner which her mother would approve of, even though this manner no longer fits her self-conception or her life-style. Everyone in the group acts out, moves in a way they believe their mother would wish. I found myself on my knees, bending down, gesturing, imploring, drawing the attention of the adult by clowning, by quick, sharp movements, by giggling, by anxious, questioning, pleading looks. I did not act any such role or scene from memory; I did not consciously attempt to summarize what I believed my mother had wanted me to be. I let my body respond to a relationship, and it summarized its essence; my smallness, submission, the intense need to get approval by any means.

The other members of the group showed very different reactions to the same request. P. almost knocked herself out by being efficient, quick and useful. B. walked through the studio demurely like a nun. A. went up smiling to everyone but saw no one. E. was uncertain if she could move at all and seemed confused. We all felt that we acted out something that had not been imparted to us verbally; what we did enact was for some of us in direct opposition to what we had been taught. A great deal of sadness came with my realization of the barrenness of this relationship to my mother and later, anger.

Anger caused us more trouble in acting out than anything else; perhaps, I should rather say rage. What is so frightening is not only the realization of one's destructiveness and one's fear of retaliation, but also the terror of losing control and of never regaining it. Let me illustrate. I disliked myself worse when I felt in myself reactions, motions, belief patterns, which, consciously, I rejected years ago. They are residues of my mother's influence upon me that I experience as alien. I should add that some of my mother's *traits* in me do not provoke such self-dislike. I demonstrated to J. a childhood day when I was ill and my mother's reaction to my illness. I was the child in pain; I was the mother calming down the child. I stopped the acting-out petrified to go on. I felt I was entering a terrible darkness that I could not tolerate. J. told me that she would go into the darkness with me. Her words felt like the hand of my brother to whom I had clung when small and frightened.

I reenacted the scene and this time *played* it through. When the mother admonished the child to be quiet and not to make a fuss, the child stopped crying and went rigid. The mother continued saying: "See, there is not much the matter with you, you are quiet now." I felt the child get up and hit out at the mother, hitting to kill. Beating and trampling about, I saw a bloody body; as this image came, I felt sick with fear and collapsed sobbing. J. held me in a manner that conveyed to me that she believed the reality of my feelings, the pain, the rage, the fear and the grief. She was not afraid of these feelings in me, hence not afraid of losing control. Since this was so, I could let her take care of me.

It does not really matter whether or not this incident constitutes a memory of an event that happened—namely the child pleads for help, the adult denies the plea and hence the child's feelings, the child believes that in her rage over the denial she has killed her mother. What does matter is that this scene showed the essence of the child's relationship to her mother; a denial of emotion and its reality on the part of the mother; a cutting off of emotions and an underlying rage that is perceived as omnipotent by the child. It does matter that J. believed the emotions, accepted them as real and was not afraid of losing control. She provided me with the consolation and courage that my brother had given me, a help I could accept in the initial stages of the scene.

In this reenactment I lived through a conviction deeply engrained and inaccessible to consciousness, namely that feeling kills, all feeling. Rationally, I knew, of course, that this was not the case. It was this conviction that at times made me cold, intellectual, uneasy, fearful, and distrustful of all feeling. In motion and gesture this conviction appeared as a guardedness and a lack of spontaneity which I recognized as an exaggeration of my mother's. In reliving the situation of mother and child, I saw not only what went wrong in the first patterning but also what is possible as a new patterning. And this, it seems to me, is truly redemption from the past into a richer present.

There were times in dance therapy when I simply could not maintain an emotion long enough in motion. I saw a figure another patient had done in clay. It was a woman about to vomit, lumps rising from her stomach up to her throat. Rough though it was, the figure was memorably expressive. J. suggested that I work out some feelings in clay, that I take a big piece of clay and work out some anger. A few days later I put on an old hospital gown in the occupational therapy room. I. the teacher, gave me a piece of clay and told me to start pounding at it. I started pounding; the clay shaped into a ball, a cylinder, a human body. I shaped out a head, drew out arms from the mass of the body and then legs. A sitting figure emerged with a body that seemed immense; a strong back, protruding belly and large breasts. Only once before in my life, I experienced such exultation in an activity, in its rightness for me. This same feeling overwhelmed me in molding this figure; I hardly noticed the other patients or the teacher.

Only as I was completing the figure and working out detail, I became aware of the pleasure of the teacher in my absorption. The first figure complete, all stood around admiring it, hugging each other, proud like children at a task well done, eager to go on to the next. I took a smaller piece of clay, thinking that I would do a woman lying down, a woman half human, half animal, a mermaid. The upper body finished, the rest of the figure did not assume shape as I had visualized. I had meant it to be a cold but peaceful figure. I found that the back was better arched, the mermaid's tail shaped into legs spread, the head bent back, the body tense, the mouth gaping. This way the figure felt right.

As the other patients and the teacher were watching me, I felt some embarrassment at the sensuousness of the figure in its agony. One patient remarked "She is obscene." I realized that this was

not so for me; if the forthrightness of my figure bothered someone, that was their trouble. I was afraid that I might be laughed
at for lack of skill, for the very force with which my figures expressed themselves. Approval from teacher, therapist and fellow
patients removed such fears.

On my way home that day I picked up a bag of clay. Looking at
trees and rocks while driving past, I saw the shapes that were
hidden in them. I remembered my favorite game as a child, to
look at blocks of wood and to see what could be made from
them: toys, dolls, animals, ships, furniture, airplanes. That evening I made another figure; but working alone was not as rewarding as it had been that afternoon. I needed the sense of
participation of the class. For some time I found that I did my
most satisfying work during the clay therapy hours. Only gradually I learned to work by myself, to do without immediate approval and participation by others.

At first I understood the meaning of my figures only weeks
after I made them. The immense women with small, ineffective
arms and legs to my teacher and to my therapist were immediately recognizable as my mother; the agonized woman, which started as mermaid, myself. I was sure to fail not only in expressive-
ness but also in being absorbed in the process of working when I
tried a subject matter, such as *the mermaid* and did not let myself be guided by the emotion that needed expression.

Working with clay was the exact reversal of my usual experience
of the world, which had been observation, evaluation, planning,
action. Rather I let *my hands express what I felt at the time.* It
was only gradually that I learned to understand and to read
what they expressed. This realization came most forcefully when
I made a mask in clay. As I looked at the emerging face I recognized a powerfully angry face; I burst out in tears of fright, but I
felt that fright was not all I experienced at that moment. I made
another face which, though more violently angry, no longer
frightened me. I tried still another which looked grieving and
a last which was gentle and sad. Thus, gradually, as I shaped
the clay, I felt which emotion was predominant and wanted to
be expressed.

There were times when I could not fully explore expression

in clay and needed to transform the incomplete feeling back into motion in dance therapy. A clay figure stretched out was expressive enough, but I felt uneasy about its discomfort. In dance therapy, as I stretched myself into the position of the figure, I felt an almost intolerable tension, as if I wanted to snap shut. I realized I was stretching against resistance toward being open; for stretching means to stretch only toward one goal, to be open to it and unguarded toward the total environment. I was tense with discomfort because I feared such total commitment and its attendant unguardedness.

When I wanted to explore one posture and its emotion more fully, clay became less and less satisfactory as a medium. I wanted a medium which would not break as easily, would be more resilient and allow for more flexibility in motion. I also wanted to prolong the actual process of working on a figure to fully feel its emotional significance. Wood seemed the right choice. My basic ideas for a figure come from emotions that occupy me, but which I do not feel through and through. I try out different movements in dance to experience what feels right. I look at blocks of wood to visualize if they are right for the kind of motion I have in mind. When I settle on a piece of wood the rough shape is there.

The first task is to get the approximate shape, a tedious task that is made easier by chiselling off in the round, by stopping frequently and assuming and feeling the body position of the figure (I could not work out, say the head, and then proceed to neck and shoulders). In this manner, even when the figure's position is recognizable to no one else, it is there for me; after a few hours of work it can no longer be changed. I once tried to change a figure turning on its hips to a straight, head-on position. Even though I had more than enough wood to make such a change, even though I could draw the figure straight-on, the image of the first figure was so strongly associated with this piece of wood, that I could not make the change.

Once the figure assumes its rough shape, it is hard to stop working. Absorption in the process is such that I forget time. Certainly, I often interrupt the chiselling in order to look at the figure, and to assume the figure's position to feel if the figure reflects the feeling; but such interruptions are part of the process and the most rewarding part. There is joy in the feeling that the figure assumes its right shape; there is surprise at a detail of expression which I had not visualized earlier and which suddenly is there.

For instance, in the figure I call the sky-lifter, I wanted a serious but graceful face. For a long time the face was much too heavy. With a few cuts, it looked too old. Finally, shaping the nose and making its root narrow, an almost Grecian face emerged. Unfortunately, I wanted to improve it and took away some of the fullness of the cheeks. Thus I ended up with a face more serious than I wanted it to be. Nevertheless, when the figure was finished, the expression of the face harmonized with the rest of her body. The finishing of a figure is also an exploration of possibilities of expression and it may happen that one possibility is chosen which does not seem right at the time but fits in the end.

As in working with clay so, too, with wood I like to explore the potentialities of a figure in dance; I like to take it with me to have friends see it and give me their reactions, in short, to share its growth. At this point in time, ideas for figures come from these sources: my own memory (figure of two children), a position in dance that contains a powerful emotion that I want to feel until I have expressed it (the pleading woman) or the observation of other patients whose *feeling position* I have empathy for.

An example of the latter is my best figure to date which I call the sorrowful woman. One evening several months ago, J. ran out of the group held at Dr. C.'s house. A few minutes later we found her lying out on the lawn, sobbing and convulsed. We brought her into the house where she dropped to the floor near the door. She was doubled over, her body resting on her legs, she looked as if she were broken in half. She did not respond to Dr. C.'s speaking for a long time, but then slowly her body arched upwards, her head half-turned from the crouching position to look at Dr. C. When I first found a block of Bulbinga wood it looked right for a figure folded into herself with her head peeking forth at the observer. As I began working, the wood grain suggested a kneeling position; the body's attitude was that of a woman raising herself up and gazing out with head still bent. The entire therapy

group participated in the making of the figure; we talked as I
chiselled, C. and I. made suggestions as to the position of the arms,
J. helped me clean out some hard-to-get-to creases. Everyone held
her to allow me to chisel out spots I would not have reached without better bracing than I now have.

Let me summarize: In the last few years I have learned to express my emotions in a way that is meaningful to me and to my
friends. As the art work gave clearer expression to my emotions,
I became more comfortable with myself. My life is taking on a
new shape, I am beginning to know what I need and I feel
surer of the ways to satisfy my needs. The need to dull emotions
by alcohol disappeared. Expression of emotion is not restricted
to working through a medium: clay, wood, or words; it is not a
substitute for relationships to others. I can equally well express
emotions through touch or words, for I have gained the assurance that whatever expresses me honestly is acceptable. Sculp-
ture or a piece of writing are merely more durable and they may
reach more people.

Some points might be made concerning such therapy and the
role of the therapists involved. Above all it is important that
they (occupational therapists as well as psychotherapist) are
not afraid of regression. If the patient cries or shouts, his emotions should be accepted; he should be encouraged to explore
them further and not be calmed down. All media, dance, music,
poetry, the visual arts should be made available so that the patient can explore which will satisfy his needs best.

It may be that for some time the patient does not show interest in any of these activities. He should nevertheless be encouraged to attend such activities regularly. Art activities should not
be regarded as past-times and they should never be mere handi-
work such as the making of paper flowers or the copying of designs. The art therapist should discourage imitation and should
encourage the patient to express what he feels.

In the beginning, a free medium such as clay may work best.
The request should not be to make an ashtray, an animal, or a
man but rather to give shape to what the patient feels; pound,
twist, caress the clay and see what happens. Any honest expression of emotion should be welcomed—technical skill or semblance

to a real object can be discouraged safely. If the patient likes the medium, he will acquire what technique he needs himself through books or regular art classes.

The art therapist need not be a person trained in artistic skills. It is best if she is a patient with artistic inclinations who is a little further along in her therapy—she has been there, she knows what mental illness feels like, she can encourage expression, she is not afraid of emotion. It is wise not to ask the patient to pursue a skill he had before therapy. If I had tried writing as a medium of expression, I could not have done anything with it, it had ceased to help me express myself; know-how and long habit had removed feeling expression from it.

Finally, it is important that several patients share an art activity, explore the possibility of new media, and share the enjoyment of their new discovery. An analogy with a supportive family describes the situation best; the therapists as parents encourage emotional expression and provide means for such expression; fellow patients like siblings participate in and enjoy together a common task. All members of the family support the achievements of each individual.

To return to the theories of Freud mentioned at the beginning of this essay concerning regression, fantasy, and sublimation. It seems to me that by regression new possibilities of expressing emotion are opened up. Regression to child-like openness is a necessary step and a positive one in therapy as well as in creativity. Given media to express himself, the patient's fresh feeling will seek for an adequate form, for a projection of that feeling into reality. In this way, by projection of feeling (what else is imagination or fantasy) the patient shapes his present. The process of shaping feeling into form defines the feeling and gives a sense of achievement.

To explore the possibilities of expressing feelings in forms leads to planning within a medium, to longer spans of concentration, to a sense of continuity, to shaping a future. Defined in this manner, fantasy does not, as Freud maintains, refer only to the past and its infantile wish fulfillments, but also to a future. And this would be a future in greater harmony with the patient's real needs and emotions as an adult.

It hardly matters if one calls such fulfillment sublimation or plain satisfaction. And such satisfaction of working and enjoying has none of the heroics, of the denigration of art and the artist, of the melodrama associated with *artistic suffering* and of the theories mentioned earlier in this paper. It is fulfillment through being able to express both pain and joy, hate and love, trust and fear. Just that, nothing more, nothing less. Although the intensity of the emotion may have a role in determining the merit of the patient's art work, emotion does not make its value as a work of art. That value is a question of aesthetics, of the history of taste and art and not of psychology.[4]

BIBLIOGRAPHY

1. Menninger, Karl: *The Vital Balance*. New York, The Viking Press, 1963.
2. Freud, Sigmund: The Poet and Day-Dreaming. In Nelson, Benjamin (Ed.): *On Creativity and the Unconscious: Papers on the Psychology of Art, Literature, Love, Religion*. New York, Harper and Row, 1958, p. 49. The essay first appeared in 1908. It should be kept in mind that Freud, lover of art that he was, would have wished this statement to be read in context and would have rejected, for instance, Theodor Reik's interpretation of Freud's opinion in *Ritual*, namely that Freud meant to denigrate art as an illusion and a product of illness.
3. Hesse during 1916-17 consulted Joseph B. Lang, a disciple of C. G. Jung's. Hesse used the self-knowledge he gained through analysis in his novels of that period, foremost in *Demian* (1920). Cf. Ziolkowski, Theodor: *The Novels of Hermann Hesse: A Study in Theme and Structure*. Princeton, New Jersey, 1965.
4. This essay is dedicated to Jack Carleton, Joan Smallwood, and Isabelle Haller.

Chapter 20

THE THERAPEUTIC COMMUNITY AND THE WORKSHOP

LUBA CARLETON

COLLOQUIA, SYMPOSIA, workshops in areas of specialization be they medicine, education, history, etc., are a focus of the need to be informed in the varied areas of specialization. We felt compelled to conduct a symposium and publish the proceedings for others to gain insights from the foregoing eminent experts in this book. Along with the information and learning that was experienced at this symposium, there developed a most important ambience and tone of closeness among those who came. This tone contributed a vital quality to the symposium milieu bridging the social and professional gap with a common bond of purposeful endeavor.

Subsequently, internalized knowledge gained from this symposium was carried back to the participants' respective professions with enthusiasm and provocative speculation and thinking. Reflecting upon the reasons for this tone, we must backtrack perhaps to a time two years prior to the workshop. We should like you, the reader, to bear with us as we retrace this happening and relate some back history.

My husband, Doctor Carleton, has for many years felt that mental health organizations and societies characteristically benefit the members of the *Charity Community* more than they benefit the recipients and patients of these services. The reasons are multitudinous, but basically those who are actively part of the formation and participation of a group activity are involved, and subsequently have a vested interest; whereas the patient in need of treatment generally is an isolated recipient of aid offered by others. Due to this orientation, and due to the need in the psychiatric practice at that time, the Santa Barbara Psychiatric Foundation evolved. Its birth came at the time when a particular patient released from a hospital needed a place to reside for a short period. Her home was one hundred miles from the office, while her therapeutic program called for intensive follow-up therapy. The patient moved into our social worker's apartment. She needed a place to live before returning home and assuming family responsibilities. Problems of everyday living arose, and both persons became intensely involved. They were able to solve their situational obstacles much of the time. Some difficulties arose that were beyond their capabilities and they turned for assistance and support to our clinic staff.

As more patients were released from the hospital, they also wished to reside at our *half-way house* (termed as such in want of a better name). Elaine's, the social worker's, apartment was overcrowded and we needed a larger facility. We also decided to give the residence some structure. Elaine was paid for time spent with the patients. Doctor Carleton undertook the responsibility for the rent, paid for staple supplies, and a weekly cleaning crew with the expectation that reimbursement would come later. The residents were to be charged a nominal fee for lodging and food.

After some time, many questions needed answers: How many patients could reside together at one time? What kind of people should reside together? What ages would be compatible? We invited interested people to attend a meeting and discuss these problems. At that first meeting, there were approximately twenty patients and their spouses, three psychiatrists and their wives, some hospital volunteers, nurses, and aides from the psychiatric unit at the local hospital. This group met at our home.

The group collectively decided to set a low fee for food and lodging; $180.00 per month so that those in need could utilize the facility. In addition, the group agreed that those who were to live there must either be employed full time or attend school. They were not to be encouraged to sit about and become useless to themselves and perhaps, in this way, nourish their emotional problems. The meeting culminated with the group's decision to form a foundation and to apply for the status of a nonprofit organization. This the group subsequently did, and today it is known as the Santa Barbara Psychiatric Foundation.

Within a matter of two weeks, Elaine found a house suitable to be a half-way house. It was badly in want of repair and paint; however, since it was just three blocks from the office and five blocks from the hospital, it was an ideal location. The rent was reasonable at $225.00 per month. The space was adequate; it had three bedrooms upstairs and a living room, kitchen, and bedroom on the first floor. A lease was signed and the evolving community set about making this new facility a home. Committees were formed; paint crews gathered; sewing groups to make curtains met and worked together; donations of furniture and household items were solicited. Within one week, the house was ready for its new family. Truly, this was the beginning of the extended family and community feeling that lives today among members of the Santa Barbara Psychiatric Foundation.

From this active beginning, members, friends, and new patients spontaneously gathered to be with one another motivated by individual wants and needs. Our potting wheel, along with clay and wood block carving, was installed in the downstairs bedroom. The foundation meetings were held at the house as well as spontaneous gatherings. No one who needed help was left alone. At times, an individual might be frightened and stay awake all night but someone was always close-by to help weather these periods.

Elaine stayed at the half-way house for one year and under her supervision, a structured tone was set. After a year she felt it was time to leave. The tone still prevailed and the new patients were now learning how to live together from the older residents. It was feared that following Elaine's absence, the house might not operate successfully, but such has not been the case. If a situational obstacle occurs, the residents call on other foundation members to help them. With each such interaction, a closer relationship evolves and self-determination and positive communication are reenforced. With each new resident the house tone changes slightly to meet the needs and personality of the new member, but the prevailing feeling of openness, respect, and closeness permeates and remains.

About the time of the emergence of the Santa Barbara Psychiatric Foundation, we felt a need to sponsor a symposium

which was to be called *Collaboration for Mental Health*. Dr.
Bierer agreed to come from England as a part of the International
Association for Social Psychiatry's plan to participate in world-
wide symposia of this nature. As we know today, it is difficult, actually impossible, to remain apart and isolated from other disciplines. As people today are in search of interpersonal closeness
and understanding, evidenced by encounter groups, university
extension classes, dance groups, adult recreation groups, etc.,
so, too, are diversified professions seeking relatedness. No longer can we remain apart and independent of each other as in the
past.

The Protestant Ethic of *hard work and thrift* is now functionally insufficient. Today, because of the diversities in technological
and communication media and because of specialization in each
field of the professions and work forces, we are much in need of
each other. We rely on each other for knowledge outside our specific fields; we rely on each for worldly goods outside our professions. We now have an interdependence that is so vital, we cannot exist and function without our neighbors.

We invited people from different disciplines. Each person, we
hoped, would learn and gain knowledge from the other. Each
could utilize the different emphases and know-how to broaden
his scope. We invited urban planners, psychiatrists, statesmen,
counselors, etc.

Members of the foundation became an integral part of the
symposium, first by assisting with the mechanics, but later in
ways which involved the personal and social interactional aspects
of the conference. The symposium gradually became theirs. They
decided to organize small luncheon groups of ten to twelve
people. Santa Barbara residents were asked to donate their houses
for the luncheons. Members of the Foundation were to host. A
tone of fulfilled expectation prevailed and foundation members
began to interact with the *well community* and relate at a peer
level. They truly were spiraling outward in breadth and depth.

Foundation members (mostly patients) handled the registration and welcoming tables. The feelings of closeness and *together-
ness* merged and became apparent. Further, they extended an

open invitation to all to visit their half-way house. They served punch, coffee and cookies. Approximately fifty people responded. These experiences and interactions contributed greatly to the workshop's success.

The ambience prevailed at the symposium and when it ended, there was a feeling of exhilaration. Friendships had developed and ideas were exchanged. There was also sadness that the workshop was over, also a part of a real experience.

INDEX

335